HAMLYN ALL COLOUR
SLIMMING COOKBOOK

HAMLYN ALL COLOUR
SLIMMING
COOKBOOK

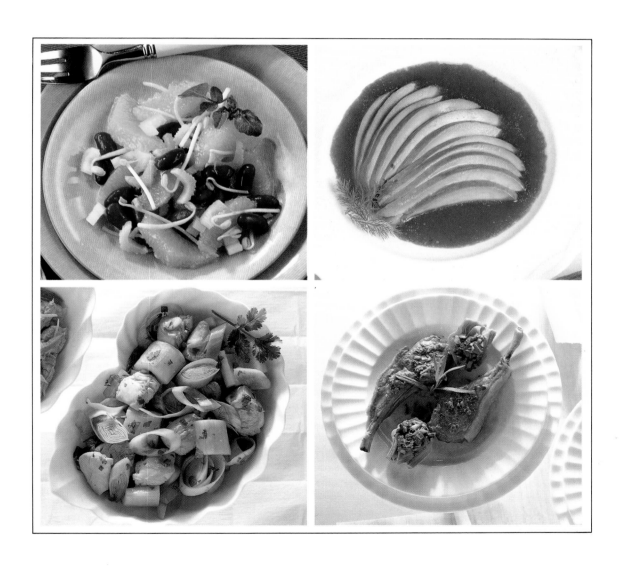

HAMLYN

Front cover shows, clockwise from top right:
Spiced Carrot Soup (1), *Spiced Pears* (229), *Lemon and Limeade*
(261), *Plaice with Cucumber* (49)

Title page and back cover show, clockwise from top right:
Avocado with Raspberry Vinaigrette (25), *Cutlets with Tarragon*
(97), *Chicken and Leeks* (141), *Orange Winter Salad* (181)

Published in 1990 by
The Hamlyn Publishing Group Limited
a division of the Octopus Publishing Group
Michelin House, 81 Fulham Road, London SW3 6RB

Line drawings by Gillie Newman

ISBN 0 600 57160 2

Produced by Mandarin Offset
Printed in Hong Kong

Contents

Useful Facts and Figures

Notes on metrication

In this book quantities are given in metric and Imperial measures. Exact conversion from Imperial to metric measures does not usually give very convenient working quantities and so the metric measures have been rounded off into units of 25 grams. The table below shows the recommended equivalents.

Ounces	Approx g to nearest whole figure	Recommended conversion to nearest unit of 25	Ounces	Approx g to nearest whole figure	Recommended conversion to nearest unit of 25
1	28	25	9	255	250
2	57	50	10	283	275
3	85	75	11	312	300
4	113	100	12	340	350
5	142	150	13	368	375
6	170	175	14	396	400
7	198	200	15	425	425
8	227	225	16 (1 lb)	454	450

Note: When converting quantities over 16 oz first add the appropriate figures in the centre column, then adjust to the nearest unit of 25. As a general guide, 1 kg (1000 g) equals 2.2 lb or about 2 lb 3 oz. This method of conversion gives good results in nearly all cases, although in certain pastry and cake recipes a more accurate conversion is necessary to produce a balanced recipe.

Liquid measures The millilitre has been used in this book and the following table gives a few examples.

Imperial	Approx ml to nearest whole figure	Recommended ml	Imperial	Approx ml to nearest whole figure	Recommended ml
¼	142	150 ml	1 pint	567	600 ml
½	283	300 ml	1½ pints	851	900 ml
¾	425	450 ml	1¾ pints	992	1000 ml (1 litre)

Spoon measures All spoon measures given in this book are level unless otherwise stated.

Can sizes At present, cans are marked with the exact (usually to the nearest whole number) metric equivalent of the Imperial weight of the contents, so we have followed this practice when giving can sizes.

60 ml = 2 fluid g.

Oven temperatures
The table below gives recommended equivalents.

	°C	°F	Gas Mark		°C	°F	Gas Mark
Very cool	110	225	¼	Moderately hot	190	375	5
	120	250	½		200	400	6
Cool	140	275	1	Hot	220	425	7
	150	300	2		230	450	8
Moderate	160	325	3	Very Hot	240	475	9
	180	350	4				

Notes for American and Australian users

In America the 8-fl oz measuring cup is used. In Australia metric measures are now used in conjunction with the standard 250-ml measuring cup. The Imperial pint, used in Britain and Australia, is 20 fl oz, while the American pint is 16 fl oz. It is important to remember that the Australian tablespoon differs from both the British and American tablespoons; the table below gives a comparison. The British standard tablespoon, which has been used throughout this book, holds 17.7 ml, the American 14.2 ml, and the Australian 20 ml. A teaspoon holds approximately 5 ml in all three countries.

British	American	Australian
1 teaspoon	1 teaspoon	1 teaspoon
1 tablespoon	1 tablespoon	1 tablespoon
2 tablespoons	3 tablespoons	2 tablespoons
3½ tablespoons	4 tablespoons	3 tablespoons
4 tablespoons	5 tablespoons	3½ tablespoons

An Imperial/American guide to solid and liquid measures

Imperial	American	Imperial	American
Solid measures		**Liquid measures**	
1 lb butter or margarine	2 cups	¼ pint liquid	⅔ cup liquid
1 lb flour	4 cups	½ pint	1¼ cups
1 lb granulated or caster sugar	2 cups	¾ pint	2 cups
1 lb icing sugar	3 cups	1 pint	2½ cups
8 oz rice	1 cup	1½ pints	3¾ cups
		2 pints	5 cups (2½ pints)

Note: When making any of the recipes in this book, only follow one set of measures as they are not interchangeable.

Introduction

The Hamlyn All Colour Slimming Cookbook is packed with imaginative, calorie-counted recipes to help you lose weight by following a sensible balanced diet. It is wise to consult your doctor as to the number of calories you should have every day to ensure that you lose weight safely. This depends on several factors such as sex, age, height and lifestyle.

A colour photograph illustrates each recipe, showing how visually appealing low-calorie dishes can be. You should always aim to make food look as tempting as possible since this will encourage you to develop a preference for a healthy pattern of eating. You will then find it easier to maintain your correct weight.

Even if you like to eat your main meal in the evening, it is important that you reserve some of your calorie allowance for breakfast and lunch. This also helps you to resist any temptation to nibble during the day.

Try to plan your meals in advance so that you can be sure you have the right ingredients available and do not find yourself having to eat fattening snacks. Treat this book as if it were a menu and pick out combinations of dishes that both appeal to you and total the requisite daily number of calories.

Many slimmers still need to cook meals for other people and naturally do not want to prepare different food for them. The recipes in this book have been carefully chosen so that you can enjoy the same food as your family and friends. If you decide, however, to make a dish that is relatively high in calories, offset this by not having a second course yourself or by choosing one with few calories.

While most people realize that a recipe containing a lot of double cream would be calorie-laden, they may not perhaps know that nuts, for instance, are also high in fat. Therefore the amount of calories in a particular dish may surprise you. Gram for gram, fat contains almost twice the calories of proteins and carbohydrates. Although polyunsaturated fats such as vegetable oils are now generally considered healthier than saturated fats such as cream, both are equally high in calories.

Some fat is, of course, necessary in a healthy diet, but most people tend to eat too much. By using non-stick pans you can easily reduce the amount of fat you use – or use the grill instead of the frying pan. Natural low-fat yogurt makes delicious sauces and salad dressings. You will find that many of the recipes combine fruit or vegetables with fish, meat or poultry for main course dishes, which cuts down the proportion of fat.

You should be realistic about the time it may take you to reach your target weight. It is much better to do this gradually by keeping within your daily calorie allowance rather than by skipping meals. In this way you will not only lose weight but also gain vitality.

With 268 recipes to choose from, dieting need never be dull.

Food Value Table

(In most cases, figures have been rounded up or down for ease of calculation)

Food	KJ/calorie per 25 g/1 oz or 25 ml/1 fl oz	KJ/calories per 100 g/4 oz or 120 ml/4 fl oz	Food	KJ/calorie per 25 g/1 oz or 25 ml/1 fl oz	KJ/calories per 100 g/4 oz or 120 ml/4 fl oz
Anchovies	190/45	750/180	**Cauliflower** – raw	20/5	80/20
Apples			**Celery** – raw	8/2	35/8
raw	40/10	170/40	**Cheese**		
dried	270/65	1090/260	Camembert	355/85	1420/340
juice	40/10	170/40	Cheddar	420-500/	1670-2000/
Apricots				100-120	400-480
raw	20/5	80/20	cottage	125/30	500/120
dried	210/50	840/200	curd	170/40	670/160
canned	125/30	500/120	Danish Blue	420/100	1670/400
Artichokes			Edam	355/85	1420/340
globe	20/5	80/20	Emmenthal	460/110	1840/440
Jerusalem	20/5	80/20	full fat soft	520/125	2090/500
Asparagus			Gouda	355/85	1420/340
fresh	20/5	80/20	Gruyère	500/120	2000/480
canned	12/3	50/12	Lancashire	420/100	1670/400
Aubergine – raw	20/5	80/20	Mozzarella	40095	1590/380
Avocado	270/65	1090/260	Parmesan	500/120	2000/480
Bacon – lean, no fat	270/65	1090/260	processed	380/90	1500/360
Bamboo shoots	40/10	170/40	Ricotta	290/70	1170/280
Banana	60/15	420/100	Sage Derby	460/110	1840/440
		(average size)	St Paulin	380/90	1500/360
			Stilton	540/130	2170/520
Beans – raw			**Cherries**		
French	8/2	35/8	raw	40/10	170/40
runner	20/5	80/20	canned	80/20	330/80
broad	60/15	250/60	**Chicken**		
butter	100/25	420/100	meat only, no skin	125/30	500/120
chick peas	100/25	420/100	poussin	80/20	330/80
haricot	100/25	420/100	**Chicory** – raw	12/3	50/12
red kidney	100/25	420/100	**Clementine**	40/10	210/50
Bean sprouts	16/4	65/16			(average size)
Beef			**Cod** – raw	80/20	330/80
lean, no fat	250/60	1000/240	**Cod roe** – smoked	125/30	500/120
steak	230/55	920/220	**Cornflour**	420/100	1670/400
minced	250/60	1000/240	**Courgettes** – raw	12/3	50/12
stewing	250/60	1000/240	**Crab** – boiled	145/35	585/140
Beetroot – raw	40/10	170/40	**Cranberries** – raw	16/4	65/16
Blackberries – raw	40/10	170/40	**Crayfish** – shelled	125/30	500/120
Blackcurrants – raw	40/10	170/40	**Crispbread**	380-420/	1500-1670/
Bread				90-100	360-400
wholemeal	250/60	1000/240	**Cucumber** – raw	12/3	50/12
Breakfast cereals	380-440/	1500-1700	**Damsons** – raw	40/10	170/40
	90-105	360-420	**Dates** – dried	250/60	1000/240
Bream – raw	100/25	420/100	**Duck** – meat only,		
Broad beans	60/15	250/60	no skin	250/60	1170/280
Brussels sprouts – boiled	20/5	80/20	**Egg**	each	
Butter	880/210	3510/840	(depending on size)	170-250/40-60	
Buttermilk	40/10	170/40	**Endive**	12/3	50/12
Cabbage			**Figs**		
raw	20/5	80/20	green, raw	40/10	170/40
red	20/5	80/20	dried	250/60	1000/240
Carrots					
raw	20/5	80/20			
canned	20/5	80/20			

Food	KJ/calorie per 25 g/1 oz or 25 ml/1 fl oz	KJ/calories per 100 g/4 oz or 120 ml/4 fl oz
Flour		
plain	420/100	1670/400
wholemeal	400/95	1590/380
Fruit juices		
apple	40/10	170/40
grape	80/20	330/80
grapefruit, unsweetened	40/10	170/40
lemon	8/2	35/8
orange, unsweetened	40/10	170/40
pineapple, unsweetened	60/15	250/60
Gelatine	400/95	1590/380
Gooseberries	20-40/5-10	80-170/20-40
Grapes	80/20	330/80
Grapefruit – fresh	12/3	50/12
		(½ portion)
Greengage – raw	60/15	250/60
Haddock		
fresh	80/20	330/80
smoked	80/20	330/80
Hake	80/20	330/80
Halibut	100/25	420/100
Honey	330/80	
Ice cream	190/45	750/180
Jam	310/75	1250300
Jelly – made with cubes	80/20	330/80
Kipper	330/80	1340/320
Lamb – lean, raw	210-290/ 50-70	840-1170/ 200-280
Leeks	20/5	80/20
Lemon – raw		20/5
		(average size)
Lentils – boiled	125/30	500/120
Lettuce	12/3	50/12
Low-fat spread	420/100	1670/400
Lychees – raw	80/20	330/80
Macaroni – raw	420/100	1670/400
Mackerel		
fresh	270/65	1000/240
smoked	380/90	1500/360
Margarine	920/220	3680/880
Marrow	12/3	50/12
Melon	20/5	80/20
Milk, cow's		
one pint	80/20	330/80
sterilized	80/20	330/80
long life	80/20	330/80
skimmed liquid	40/10	170/40
powdered skimmed	420/100	1670/400
Mushrooms	8/2	35/8
Nectarines – raw	60/15	250/60
		(average size)
Nuts		
almonds	670/160	2680/640
brazils	730/175	2930/700
cashews	650/155	2590/620
hazelnuts	460/110	1840/440
peanuts	670/160	2680/640
walnuts	630/150	2500/600
Oatmeal – raw	480/115	1920/460
Offal		
brain, boiled	170/40	670/160
heart, raw	145/35	585/140

Food	KJ/calorie per 25 g/1 oz or 25 ml/1 fl oz	KJ/calories per 100 g/4 oz or 120 ml/4 fl oz
kidney, raw	100/25	420/100
liver, raw	190/45	750/180
sweetbread, raw	170/40	670/160
tongue	230/55	920/220
Olives	100/25	420/100
Olive oil	1045/250	4200/1000
Onions	20/5	80/30
Oranges	40/10	170/40
Parsnips	60/50	250/60
Peaches – fresh	40/10	170/40
Peanut butter	730/175	2930/700
Pearl barley – raw	420/100	1670/400
Pears – fresh	60/15	250/60
Peas	80/20	330/80
Pheasant	250/60	1000/240
Pineapple – fresh	60/15	250/60
Pigeon	270/65	1090/260
Plaice	100/25	420/100
Plums – raw	40/10	170/40
Pork – lean, raw	210/50	840/200
Potatoes		
boiled	100/25	420/100
mashed	145/35	585/140
baked	125/30	500/120
roast	190/45	750/180
chips	290/70	1170/280
Prunes, dried	170/40	670/160
Rabbit – raw	145/35	585/140
Radishes	20/5	80/20
Raisins	290/70	1170/280
Raspberries	20/5	80/20
Redcurrants – raw	20/5	80/20
Rhubarb – raw	8/2	35/8
Rice – raw	440/105	1760/420
Salmon	210/540	840/200
Sardines – drained	250/60	1000/240
		(average size)
Skate	80/20	330/80
Sole	80/20	330/80
Soya beans	480/115	1920/460
Spinach	20/5	80/20
Spring greens	12/3	40/10
Spring onions	20/5	80/20
Strawberries	40/10	170/40
Sugar	460/110	1840/440
Sultanas	290/70	1170/280
Sweetcorn – canned	80/20	330/80
Tagliatelle	40/105	1760/420
Tangerine – fresh	20/5	80/20
Tomatoes – raw	20/5	80/20
Tuna – no oil	290/70	1170/280
Turbot – raw	100/25	420/100
Turkey – no skin	125/30	500/120
Turnips	20/5	80/20
Veal – lean, no fat	125/30	500/120
Vegetable oils	1045/250	4200/1000
Whiting – raw	100/25	420/100
Winkles	20/5	60/15
Yeast		
fresh	60/15	250/60
dried	210/50	840/200
Yeast extract	210/50	840/200

Soups

Soup is not only an excellent starter but it can also make a satisfying snack meal for slimmers. Choose from the wide variety of soups, from the sophisticated Avgolemono to the substantial Hearty Fish Soup, featured in this chapter. Try making other nourishing fish soups, such as Fish and Leek, to add variety to your diet. Unusual combinations of herbs, spices and vegetables are used to create deliciously different soups such as Marrow and Dill. Refreshing iced soups are ideal for light summer lunches, served with a tangy salad; they also provide an elegant first course for a dinner party.

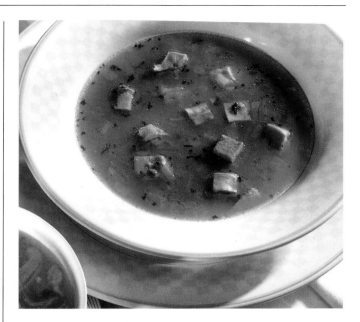

1 | Spiced Carrot Soup

Preparation time
15 minutes

Cooking time
25 minutes

Serves 4

Calories
91 per portion

You will need
1 onion, finely chopped
1 tablespoon olive oil
450 g/1 lb carrots, peeled and
    roughly chopped
1 slice fresh root ginger, 5 mm/
    ¼ inch thick
generous pinch of mixed spice
1 teaspoon grated orange rind
600 ml/1 pint chicken stock
300 ml/½ pint skimmed milk
1 teaspoon chopped fresh
    coriander

For the garnish
carrot slivers
fresh coriander sprigs

Fry the onion gently in the oil for 3 minutes; add the carrots and fry together for a further 2-3 minutes. Squeeze the fresh ginger in a garlic press and add the juice to the vegetables; add the mixed spice, orange rind, stock, skimmed milk and chopped coriander. Cover, bring to the boil and simmer gently for about 20 minutes, until the carrots are tender.

Blend the soup in a liquidizer until smooth. Reheat the soup, adjusting the consistency with a little extra stock if desired, then ladle into warmed soup bowls and garnish with the carrot slivers and coriander sprigs.

2 | Herby Chicken Soup

Preparation time
15 minutes

Cooking time
10-15 minutes

Serves 4

Calories
87 per portion

You will need
2 teaspoons oil
1 onion, finely chopped
175 g/6 oz cooked chicken,
    chopped
900 ml/1½ pints boiling water
1 tablespoon soy sauce
small pinch of dried sage
small pinch of ground cinnamon
½ small garlic clove, crushed
2 tablespoons skimmed milk
    powder
2 tablespoons cold water
1 tablespoon chopped parsley
pepper

Heat the oil in a saucepan, add the onion and fry for 3 minutes, stirring, until transparent. Add the chicken, water, soy sauce, sage, cinnamon and garlic. Bring to the boil, then simmer for 5 minutes.

Combine the milk powder with the water. Stir a little of the soup into the milk, then slowly add this mixture to the pan, stirring constantly over a gentle heat. Add the parsley and pepper to taste.

Cook's Tip

Fresh root ginger is available in some large supermarkets and in street markets in areas with a cosmopolitan population. If you do not have a garlic press, use a pestle and mortar to extract as much juice as possible.

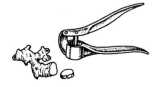

Cook's Tip

Take care not to let the soup boil after the milk has been added or it may curdle. If you would like a slightly richer soup, use semi-skimmed fresh milk instead of the reconstituted powder.

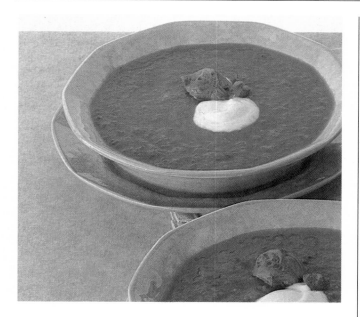

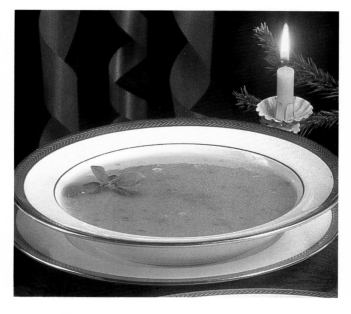

3 | *Pepper and Tomato Soup*

Preparation time
20 minutes

Cooking time
40 minutes

Serves 4

Calories
58 per portion

You will need
2 teaspoons vegetable oil
1 onion, finely chopped
2 green peppers, seeded and
    chopped
1 garlic clove, crushed
450 g/1 lb tomatoes, peeled and
    chopped
1 tablespoon tomato purée
750 ml/1¼ pints vegetable stock
1 teaspoon dried basil
salt and pepper

For the garnish
2 tablespoons natural low-fat
    yogurt
fresh basil leaves

Heat the oil in a pan and fry the onion until soft. Add the green pepper and cook for 2 minutes. Stir in the garlic, tomatoes, tomato purée, stock, basil, salt and pepper. Bring to the boil, cover and simmer for 30 minutes. Allow to cool slightly. Put in a liquidizer or food processor and work to a purée.

Before serving, reheat and check the seasoning. Pour into warmed bowls and garnish with the yogurt and basil.

4 | *Carrot and Sage Soup*

Preparation time
15 minutes

Cooking time
50 minutes

Serves 6

Calories
71 per portion

You will need
25 g/1 oz butter
1 large onion, finely chopped
750 g/1 ½ lb carrots, finely sliced
1.75 litres/3 pints stock
salt and pepper
1 tablespoon chopped fresh sage
fresh sage sprigs, to garnish
    (optional)

Melt the butter in a large heavy-based pan and gently fry the onion until transparent, then add the carrots and stock. Season with salt and pepper. Bring to the boil and simmer, uncovered, for about 30 minutes.

Liquidize the soup, then return to the pan and add the chopped sage. Bring to the boil and simmer for another 15 minutes. Serve, garnished with sage sprigs, if using.

Cook's Tip

Buy tomato purée in tubes. When opened, these can be stored in a refrigerator for several weeks. To remove the last scrap of purée from the tube, remove the cap and slowly roll a rolling pin over the tube.

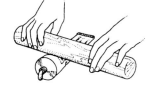

Cook's Tip

Fresh sage is usually available in large supermarkets during the winter months. If you cannot find any, dried sage may be used instead. Soak the leaves first in a tablespoon of warmed dry white wine for about 20 minutes.

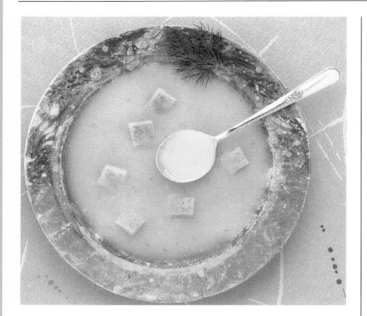

5 | Jerusalem Artichoke Soup

Preparation time
20 minutes

Cooking time
35 minutes

Serves 4

Calories
138 per portion

You will need
500 g/1 ¼ lb Jerusalem
   artichokes, scraped clean
3 tablespoons lemon juice
1 tablespoon sunflower oil
900 ml/1 ½ pints marrowbone or
   chicken stock
1 teaspoon dried dill
½ teaspoon sugar
salt and pepper

For the lemon croûtons
4 slices crustless bread
1 tablespoon lemon juice

Chop the artichokes into small pieces, sprinkling them liberally with lemon juice as you work.

Heat the oil and add the artichokes, stir well. Cover and sweat over a gentle heat for 1-2 minutes. Pour on the stock, bring to the boil, cover and simmer for about 30 minutes. Liquidize the artichokes, adding the dried dill and sugar, then rub through a sieve and return to the pan. Reheat, and add salt and pepper to taste.

To make the lemon croûtons, brush both sides of the slices of bread with lemon juice and toast until lightly coloured on both sides. Cut into cubes.

Serve the soup, garnished with the croûtons.

6 | Celery and Almond Soup

Preparation time
15 minutes

Cooking time
15 minutes

Serves 4

Calories
156 per portion

You will need
1 small onion, finely chopped
6 celery sticks, finely chopped
1 tablespoon coarsely chopped
   parsley
1 teaspoon dill seed
50 g/2 oz blanched almonds
300 ml/½ pint chicken stock
300 ml/½ pint skimmed milk
3 tablespoons natural low-fat
   yogurt
1 egg yolk
1 tablespoon toasted flaked
   almonds, to garnish

Put the onion, celery, parsley, dill seed, almonds, stock and milk into a saucepan; bring to the boil and simmer gently for about 12 minutes until the vegetables are tender.

Blend the soup in a liquidizer until smooth. Return to a clean saucepan. Beat the yogurt with the egg yolk and stir into the soup. Reheat the soup gently; do not allow it to boil.

Ladle into small bowls and sprinkle with the toasted almonds.

Cook's Tip

Jerusalem artichokes are not related to globe artichokes – they are members of the sunflower family which is why sunflower oil is the best one to use. The lemon juice will help to prevent the artichokes from discolouring.

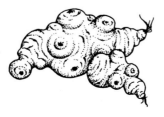

Cook's Tip

To toast the almonds, put them in a thick-based frying pan over a low heat for 2-3 minutes, stirring constantly. Do not use any fat as the oil in the nuts will prevent them sticking to the pan.

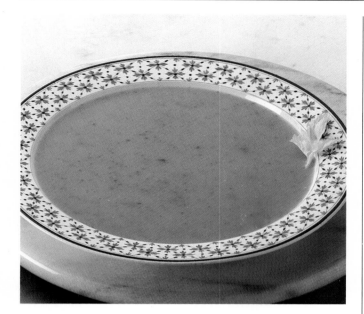

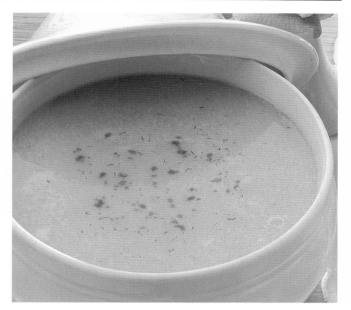

7 | Tomato and Watercress Soup

Preparation time
15 minutes

Cooking time
30 minutes

Serves 4

Calories
46 per portion

You will need
450 g/1 lb tomatoes, peeled and
    chopped
2 tablespoons fine oatmeal
1 teaspoon paprika
1 teaspoon dried oregano
2 tablespoons chopped mint
2 bay leaves
1 blade of mace
6 peppercorns
4-6 parsley stalks
2 tablespoons celery leaves
750 ml/1¼ pints chicken stock
1 bunch watercress sprigs,
    trimmed
2 teaspoons lemon juice
salt and pepper
celery leaves, to garnish

Put the tomatoes into a saucepan over a moderate heat and stir in the oatmeal and paprika. When well blended, stir in the oregano and mint. Tie the bay leaves, mace, peppercorns, parsley and celery leaves in a piece of muslin and add with the stock. Stir well and bring the soup to the boil slowly, stirring constantly. Cover the pan and simmer for 20 minutes. Discard the bag of flavourings. Put the soup in a liquidizer and purée.

Return the purée to the pan. Chop the watercress, stir it into the purée with the lemon juice and season with salt and pepper. Simmer for about 3 minutes until the watercress is just tender. Garnish the soup with celery leaves and serve hot.

Cook's Tip

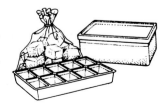

A good home-made stock is the secret of delicious soups. It is well worth making a large quantity and freezing it in different sized containers. Freeze some in ice-cube trays so that small amounts can be thawed quickly.

8 | Marrow and Dill Soup

Preparation time
15 minutes, plus
standing time

Cooking time
20 minutes

Serves 4

Calories
83 per portion

You will need
1 kg/2¼ lb marrow, peeled,
    seeded and grated
salt
1½ teaspoons oil
1½ teaspoons plain flour
1 tablespoon mild French mustard
1 tablespoon dried dill
900 ml/1½ pints chicken stock
1 tablespoon lemon juice
1 teaspoon sugar (optional)
paprika, to garnish

Put the marrow in a colander, sprinkle a little salt over and leave to stand for 20 minutes.

Heat the oil in a large saucepan, put in the marrow and sprinkle with the flour. Stir well, then cook for 1 minute, stirring all the time. Add the mustard and half the dill, stir, then pour the stock in slowly, still stirring. Cover and simmer very gently for 15-20 minutes, do not allow to boil vigorously.

For a smooth-textured soup, cool slightly, then blend in a liquidizer. Taste and adjust the seasoning, adding lemon juice and sugar as necessary. Stir in the remaining dill. Pour into warmed soup bowls, sprinkle a little paprika over each portion and serve.

Cook's Tip

For a richer soup, one teaspoonful of smetana may be placed in the bottom of each bowl before the soup is poured in. This will, of course, increase the calories per portion slightly as well.

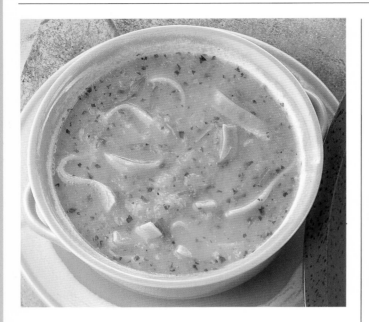

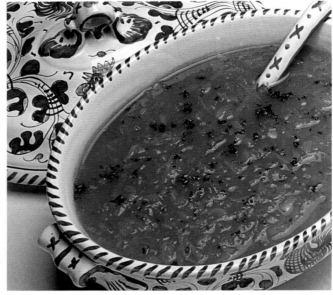

9 | Green Garden Soup

Preparation time
20 minutes

Cooking time
30-35 minutes

Serves 4

Calories
103 per portion

You will need
4 celery sticks, chopped
2 leeks, cleaned and chopped
1 bunch watercress, washed and
   chopped
1 heart of a round lettuce,
   shredded
4 spring onions, chopped
1 tablespoon chopped fresh
   tarragon
1 garlic clove, crushed
1 small head fennel, shredded
600 ml/1 pint chicken stock
300 ml/½ pint skimmed milk
salt and pepper
50 g/2 oz fine green fettucine,
   broken into short lengths

Put the celery, leeks, watercress, lettuce, spring onions, tarragon, garlic and fennel into a large saucepan; add the stock, skimmed milk and salt and pepper to taste. Simmer the soup for 20-25 minutes until all the vegetables are tender.

Blend the soup in a liquidizer until smooth. Return the soup to a clean pan and bring to the boil; add the broken fettucine and simmer for about 4 minutes, until the pasta is just tender. Serve the soup piping hot.

10 | Tomato and Carrot Soup

Preparation time
10 minutes

Cooking time
35 minutes

Serves 4

Calories
38 per portion

You will need
1 x 400-g/14-oz can tomatoes,
   chopped
2 large carrots, grated
1 small onion, finely chopped
300 ml/½ pint stock
1 teaspoon oregano
grated nutmeg
salt
1 bay leaf
1 teaspoon brown sugar
1 tablespoon chopped parsley, to
   garnish

Put the tomatoes and their juice in a saucepan. Add the carrot, onion, stock, oregano, nutmeg and salt to taste, bay leaf and sugar. Bring to the boil, stirring, cover and simmer for 30 minutes. Remove the bay leaf.

Pour the soup into a warmed tureen and sprinkle with parsley.

Cook's Tip

When cooked, fennel becomes milder and sweeter in flavour than when it is used raw in salads. It has a distinctive taste of aniseed. Available from September to April, the main crop is harvested in October and November.

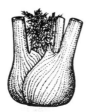

Cook's Tip

The teaspoonful of brown sugar brings out the flavour of the vegetables. Either chicken stock or, if you are a vegetarian, a stock made from root vegetables would be suitable for this economical recipe.

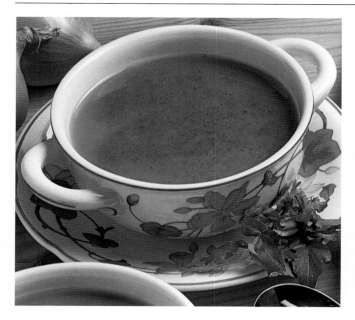

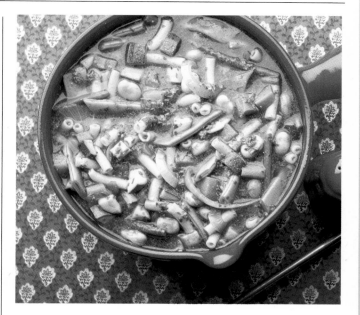

11 | Onion and Watercress Soup

Preparation time
10 minutes

Cooking time
25 minutes

Serves 4

Calories
29 per portion

You will need
1 bunch watercress
2 onions, sliced
900 ml/1½ pints light chicken
   stock
grated nutmeg
salt and pepper
40 g/1½ oz skimmed milk powder
few watercress leaves, to garnish

Wash the watercress, remove the coarse stalks and chop roughly. Put in a saucepan with the onion, stock and grated nutmeg, and salt and pepper to taste. Bring to the boil, cover and simmer for 20 minutes. Leave to cool slightly.

Put the watercress mixture in a liquidizer with the skimmed milk powder. Blend until smooth, then return to the pan. Bring to the boil, stirring, and cook for 1-2 minutes. Check the seasoning and pour into warmed bowls. Garnish with the watercress leaves.

12 | Provençal Vegetable Soup

Preparation time
30 minutes

Cooking time
30 minutes

Serves 6

Calories
219 per portion

You will need
250 g/9 oz courgettes, chopped
100 g/4 oz leeks, chopped
450 g/1 lb tomatoes, peeled and
   chopped
175 g/6 oz carrots, chopped
450 g/1 lb onions, chopped
250 g/9 oz young runner beans
250 g/9 oz French beans
250 g/9 oz broad beans, shelled
   weight
1.2 litres/2 pints veal or chicken
   stock
salt and pepper
100 g/4 oz short-cut macaroni
50 g/2 oz Parmesan cheese,
   grated, to serve

For the pesto
3 garlic cloves
9 basil sprigs
3 tablespoons olive oil

Put the vegetables in a large saucepan. Add the veal or chicken stock, and season to taste with salt and pepper. Bring to the boil, cover and simmer for 15 minutes. Add the macaroni and cook for 10-12 minutes.

Meanwhile, make the pesto. Put the garlic and basil in a mortar and pound to a paste. Add the oil, drop by drop. Remove the soup from the heat and stir in the pesto.

Ladle into a warmed tureen or individual bowls, sprinkle with Parmesan cheese and serve immediately.

Cook's Tip

Watercress is rich in vitamins and minerals. Its spicy, pungent flavour gives a piquancy to this soup. When preparing the watercress, discard any blemished or discoloured leaves. It should be used as soon as possible.

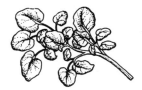

Cook's Tip

Fresh basil must be used for making the pesto. If it is unobtainable, omit the pesto and add 2 crushed garlic cloves and 1 tablespoon chopped parsley to the soup, with the stock. Alternatively, use 2-3 tablespoons prepared pesto sauce which is available in large supermarkets.

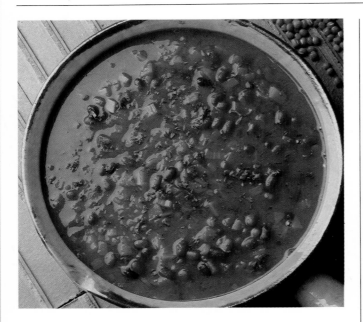

13 | Aduki Bean Soup

Preparation time
15 minutes, plus
soaking

Cooking time
1¼ hours

Serves 4

Calories
174 per portion

You will need
100 g/4 oz aduki beans
2 tablespoons oil
1 onion, chopped
1 celery stick, chopped
1 carrot, chopped
1 garlic clove, crushed
2 tomatoes, peeled and chopped
1 tablespoon tomato purée
1 bay leaf
1 teaspoon chopped thyme
900 ml/1½ pints stock or water
salt and pepper
chopped parsley

Soak the beans in cold water to cover for 3 hours; drain well.

Heat the oil in a large saucepan, add the onion, celery and carrot and cook until softened. Add the remaining ingredients, with salt and pepper to taste. Bring to the boil, boil for 10 minutes, then simmer for 1 hour.

Pour into a warmed soup tureen and sprinkle with the parsley to serve.

Cook's Tip

Aduki (or adzuki) beans have a sweet but fairly strong flavour. These tiny, dark red beans are rich in protein. They are native to Japan and are popular in Far Eastern cooking. If unobtainable, substitute kidney beans.

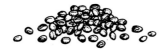

14 | Fish and Leek Soup

Preparation time
15 minutes

Cooking time
20 minutes

Serves 4

Calories
177 per portion

You will need
1 small onion, thinly sliced
1 garlic clove, crushed
2 tablespoons olive oil
2 medium leeks, cleaned and cut
    into fine strips
2 tablespoons chopped parsley
225 g/8 oz white fish fillet, cubed
300 ml/½ pint chicken stock
300 ml/½ pint skimmed milk
salt and pepper
3 tablespoons natural low-fat
    yogurt
1 egg yolk
1 tablespoon finely chopped green
    pepper, to garnish

Fry the onion and garlic gently in the olive oil for 3 minutes; add the leeks and parsley and fry for a further 3 minutes. Add the cubed fish, stock, skimmed milk and salt and pepper to taste; bring to the boil and simmer gently for 10 minutes.

Beat the yogurt and egg yolk together. Blend with a little of the hot soup and then add to the remaining soup in the pan. Heat through gently, without boiling, for 1-2 minutes.

Serve piping hot, garnished with finely chopped green pepper.

Cook's Tip

If you like a more pronounced taste of fish, replace the chicken stock with fish stock made from the skin and trimmings. This soup is substantial enough for a light meal on a winter's day.

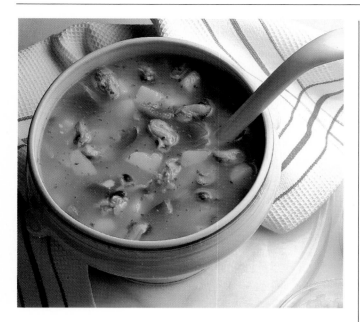

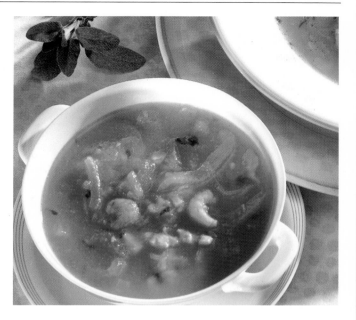

15 | Mussel Chowder

Preparation time
15 minutes

Cooking time
30 minutes

Serves 4

Calories
183 per portion

You will need
1 green pepper, seeded and
  chopped
1 small onion, chopped
350 g/12 oz potatoes, chopped
1 litre/1¾ pints fish or chicken
  stock
1 x 425-g/15-oz can shelled
  mussels, drained
salt and pepper
4 tablespoons skimmed milk
  powder
chopped parsley, to garnish

Put the pepper, onion, potatoes and stock in a large saucepan and bring to the boil. Reduce the heat, skim off the scum that rises to the surface, cover and simmer for 20 minutes.

Add the mussels and season to taste with salt and pepper, then simmer for a further 5 minutes. Cool slightly. Stir in the milk powder. Serve hot, garnished with chopped parsley.

16 | Hearty Fish Soup

Preparation time
20 minutes

Cooking time
15 minutes

Serves 4

Calories
122 per portion

You will need
1 x 175-g/6-oz portion haddock,
  fresh or frozen and thawed
1 x 175-g/6-oz portion cod, fresh or
  frozen and thawed
1 tablespoon oil
2 onions, thinly sliced
1 celery stick, finely chopped
2 garlic cloves, crushed
1 x 400-g/14-oz can chopped
  tomatoes
2 tablespoons peeled prawns
juice of ½ lemon
½ teaspoon sugar
1 tablespoon chopped parsley
3 pinches of ground bay leaves
pinch of dried thyme
generous pinch of powdered
  saffron
pepper to taste
600 ml/1 pint boiling water

Cut the fish into small pieces. Heat the oil in a saucepan, add the onion and fry for 2 minutes, without browning. Add the celery and fry for 2 minutes, stirring.

Stir in the remaining ingredients, bring to the boil, then cover and simmer for 8-10 minutes. Serve hot.

Cook's Tip

To make this chowder with fresh mussels, buy about 1.5 kg/3 lb mussels in their shells. Scrub, pulling off the beards and discarding any mussels that are open. Cook quickly in about 200 ml/7 fl oz stock for 5-6 minutes.

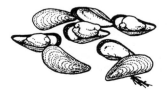

Cook's Tip

Dried bay leaves keep their flavour for a long time, stored in a screw-topped jar. Crush 2-3 leaves in a pestle and mortar which is much easier to clean than a herb mill.

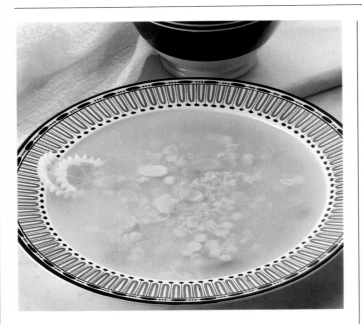

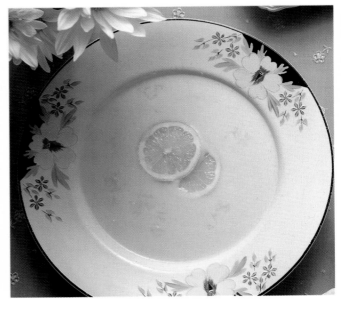

17 | *Rasan Soup*

Preparation time
15 minutes, plus
soaking

Cooking time
55 minutes

Serves 4

Calories
82 per portion

You will need
100 g/4 oz yellow split peas,
   soaked overnight and drained
1 onion, finely chopped
2 celery sticks, thinly sliced
1 small leek, trimmed and thinly
   sliced
2 teaspoons grated lemon rind
3 tablespoons lemon juice
½ teaspoon ground turmeric
2 tablespoons medium oatmeal
1 litre/1¾ pints chicken stock
salt and pepper
4 tablespoons natural low-fat
   yogurt (optional)
4 thin lemon slices, to garnish

Put the split peas, onion, celery, leek, lemon rind, lemon juice, turmeric and oatmeal into a saucepan, stir them together and pour on the stock. Bring to the boil, cover and simmer for 45 minutes. Season with salt and pepper and simmer for a further 5 minutes.

Swirl the yogurt on top, if using, and garnish the soup with the lemon slices. Serve hot.

18 | *Avgolemono*

Preparation time
10 minutes

Cooking time
25-30 minutes

Serves 4

Calories
65 per portion

You will need
1.2 litres/2 pints chicken stock
2 teaspoons finely grated lemon
   rind
1 sprig parsley
1 sprig thyme
50 g/2 oz long-grain rice
salt and pepper
2 eggs
2 tablespoons lemon juice
lemon slices, to garnish

Pour the stock into a saucepan, add the lemon rind and herbs. Bring to the boil, add the rice and a little seasoning. Reduce the heat and simmer for 20 minutes, or until the rice is tender.

Beat the eggs and lemon juice together in a bowl, whisk in a little hot, but not boiling, stock from the saucepan. Pour the egg mixture into the hot soup; simmer very gently, stirring constantly, until the soup thickens. Add any extra seasoning required, remove the sprigs of herbs and serve at once topped with lemon slices.

Cook's Tip

Turmeric not only gives a distinctive flavour to the soup but also adds colour. Madras turmeric is considered the best variety. Buy all spices in small quantities and store them in a cool dark place in screw-topped jars.

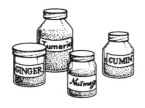

Cook's Tip

After the egg mixture has been added to the hot soup, the liquid must not be allowed to boil as the eggs may curdle. If preferred, a double saucepan can be used but this will increase the cooking time a little.

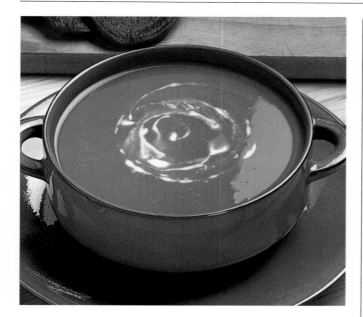

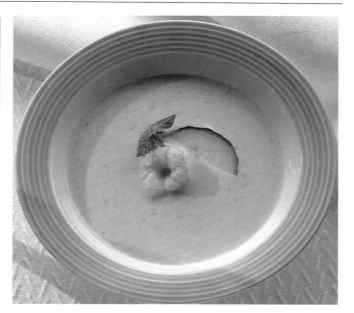

19 | Bortsch

Preparation time
20 minutes, plus
cooling

Cooking time
1¼ hours

Serves 4

Calories
91 per portion

You will need
2 teaspoons oil
1 onion, chopped
2 celery sticks, chopped
350 g/12 oz beetroot, chopped
100 g/4 oz white cabbage,
    shredded
900 ml/1½ pints stock
1 tablespoon vinegar
salt and pepper
1 bay leaf
about 3 tablespoons water
150 ml/¼ pint natural low-fat
    yogurt

Heat the oil in a saucepan, add the onion and celery and
fry until soft. Add the beetroot and cabbage, then stir in
the stock, vinegar, salt and pepper to taste, and bay leaf.
Bring to the boil, cover and simmer for 1 hour.

Leave to cool slightly, remove the bay leaf, then purée
in a liquidizer or rub through a sieve. Return to the pan,
adding just enough water to give a pouring consistency.
Check the seasoning and reheat. Pour into warmed serving bowls and stir in a little yogurt. Serve immediately.

20 | Iced Cucumber Soup

Preparation time
15 minutes, plus
chilling

Cooking time
15-20 minutes

Serves 4

Calories
203 per portion

You will need
25 g/1 oz butter
1 cucumber, chopped
2 shallots, chopped
450 ml/¾ pint semi-skimmed milk
2 garlic cloves, crushed
1 bay leaf
salt and pepper
1 tablespoon chopped mint
1 tablespoon chopped chives
250 g/9 oz prawns
5 tablespoons natural low-fat
    yogurt
3 tablespoons smetana

For the garnish
mint sprigs
cucumber slices
peeled prawns

Melt the butter in a saucepan, add the cucumber and
shallots, cover and cook gently for 5 minutes, until softened but not brown.

Add the milk, garlic, bay leaf, and salt and pepper to
taste, and simmer for 10 minutes. Remove the bay leaf.
Pour the soup into a liquidizer or food processor and work
until smooth. Pour into a soup tureen and stir in the
herbs, prawns, yogurt and smetana. Chill for 2 hours.

Garnish with mint, cucumber slices and prawns to
serve.

Cook's Tip

**If the beetroot leaves are
young and tender, they can be
used as a vegetable. Wash the
leaves carefully and boil or
steam for 10-15 minutes.
Beetroot juice can stain a
wooden chopping board so it
is wise to use a plastic one.**

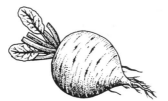

Cook's Tip

**Follow this quite rich soup
with a low-calorie main
course! Cooking the
vegetables in butter makes
the soup taste better than
using any other fat or oil.
Smetana gives a smooth
texture to this soup.**

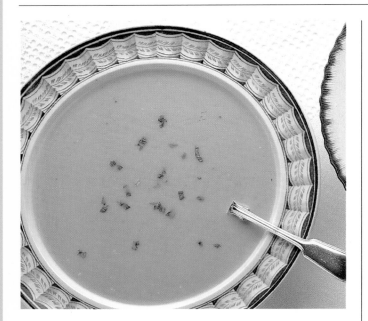

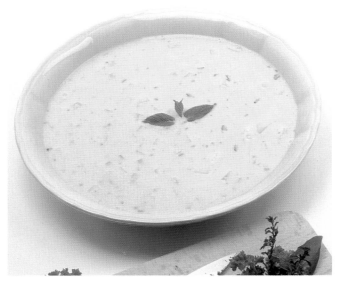

21 | *Chilled Pea Soup*

Preparation time
20 minutes, plus chilling

Cooking time
20 minutes

Serves 4

Calories
118 per portion

You will need
350 g/12 oz fresh shelled peas
225 g/8 oz potatoes, chopped
1 onion, chopped
1 large mint sprig
finely grated rind of ½ lemon
2 tablespoons lemon juice
900 ml/1½ pints chicken stock
salt and pepper
1 tablespoon chopped fresh mint, to garnish

Put the peas in a large saucepan with the potatoes, onion, mint sprig, lemon rind and juice and stock. Season with salt and pepper. Simmer, covered, for 15-20 minutes, or until the peas are tender.

Purée in a liquidizer or rub through a sieve. Set aside to cool.

Adjust the seasoning to taste and chill for 2-3 hours. Serve chilled, sprinkled with the mint.

22 | *Coriander Yogurt Soup*

Preparation time
10 minutes, plus chilling

Serves 4

Calories
83 per portion

You will need
300 ml/½ pint natural low-fat yogurt
150 ml/¼ pint tomato juice
300 ml/½ pint semi-skimmed milk
1 garlic clove, crushed
1 small cucumber, peeled and finely diced
2 tablespoons chopped fresh coriander
salt and pepper
coriander sprigs, to garnish

Put the yogurt and tomato juice in a bowl and mix together thoroughly. Stir in the milk, garlic, cucumber, most of the chopped coriander, and salt and pepper to taste. Chill for 2 hours.

Pour the soup into a tureen, and sprinkle with the remaining coriander. Garnish with coriander sprigs to serve.

Cook's Tip

If you are short of time or fresh peas are unavailable, use frozen petits pois. They will take less time to cook so add them to the other ingredients in the pan after 5-10 minutes.

Cook's Tip

Although coriander is one of the oldest herbs in cultivation, it has only recently become popular in Britain. The seeds are often used in Eastern dishes such as curry. The leaves are mildly aromatic and taste slightly of orange.

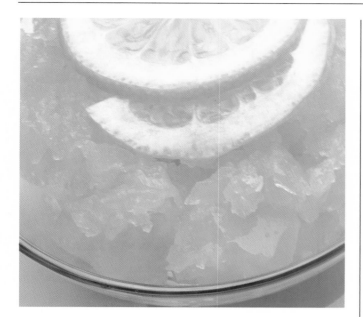

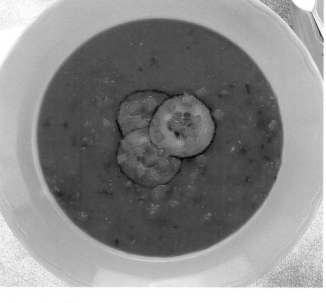

23 | Jellied Grapefruit and Cucumber Soup

Preparation time
10 minutes, plus
chilling and setting

Cooking time
10 minutes

Serves 4

Calories
67 per portion

You will need
25 g/1 oz powdered gelatine
1 litre/1 ¾ pints unsweetened
   grapefruit juice
salt and pepper
1 cucumber, peeled and grated
4 lemon slices, to garnish

Dissolve the gelatine in 3 tablespoons of the grapefruit juice over a pan of simmering water. Add the remaining grapefruit juice, season with salt and pepper and allow to cool.

As the grapefruit mixture begins to thicken, stir in the grated cucumber. Allow the mixture to set in the refrigerator for about 2 hours.

To serve, chop the jelly roughly with a sharp knife and spoon into individual glasses. Garnish with lemon slices.

24 | Gazpacho

Preparation time
25 minutes, plus
chilling

Serves 4

Calories
33 per portion

You will need
450 g/1 lb tomatoes, peeled,
   seeded and chopped
1 green pepper, seeded and
   roughly chopped
1 red pepper, seeded and roughly
   chopped
1 small onion, roughly chopped
1 large garlic clove, chopped
about 450 ml/¾ pint chicken
   stock
salt and pepper
1 tablespoon lemon juice (optional)

For the garnish
ice cubes
cucumber slices
1 tablespoon finely chopped red
   pepper

Put the tomatoes, peppers, onions, garlic and chicken stock into a liquidizer; blend until fairly smooth. Pour the blended soup into a bowl and season to taste, adding the lemon juice if necessary. Cover the soup and chill for at least 3 hours.

Ladle the chilled soup into soup bowls; add an ice cube to each one, and float cucumber slices sprinkled with a little chopped red pepper on top.

Cook's Tip

If you leave some skin on one end of the cucumber, it will be easier to hold while you are grating it. Alternatively, you could use a food processor or vary the soup by including the cucumber skin.

Cook's Tip

The easiest way to peel tomatoes is to put them in a small pan of boiling water, leave for 6-10 seconds, then lift out with a slotted spoon. When cool, make a small nick in the top of each tomato and peel off the skin.

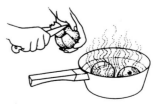

Starters

This chapter contains a truly international selection of recipes, including some from France, Italy and the Middle East. Mostly quick and easy to prepare, many of these dishes can also be served as a light meal and some are suitable for packed lunches and picnics. Seafood is always popular as a first course and Scallops with Dill and Lime and Stuffed Mussels are healthy alternatives to the traditional fish cocktails smothered in calorie-laden mayonnaise. Recipes as different as Sunshine Fruit Kebabs and Pears with Curd Cheese show how versatile fresh fruit can be in making unusual starters.

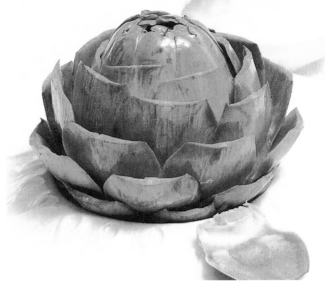

25 | Avocado with Raspberry Vinaigrette

Preparation time
15 minutes

Serves 4

Calories
127 per portion

You will need
2 avocados, halved and stoned
1 tablespoon lemon juice
100 g/4 oz raspberries
2 tablespoons olive oil
1 tablespoon wine vinegar
½ teaspoon clear honey
salt and pepper
fennel leaves, to garnish (optional)

Peel each avocado half and place cut side down on a serving plate. Slice through the avocados lengthways, then separate the slices slightly. Brush lightly with the lemon juice.

Press the raspberries through a nylon sieve to remove the seeds, then mix with the oil, vinegar, honey and salt and pepper to taste. Spoon a little around each avocado and serve immediately, garnished with fennel if liked.

26 | Globe Artichokes

Preparation time
25 minutes, plus cooling

Cooking time
25-40 minutes

Serves 4

Calories
71 per portion

You will need
4 globe artichokes
3 tablespoons light French dressing (see recipe 181)

Pull off the tough outer leaves from each artichoke and cut off the stalks. The artichokes should stand upright when cooked. The tops of the leaves can be trimmed with a pair of kitchen scissors but this is not essential.

Wash the artichokes in cold water, then put into a large pan of boiling salted water to cover and cook until tender. The cooking time varies considerably; small young artichokes need about 25 minutes while large mature artichokes can take 35-40 minutes.

Remove from the water and drain thoroughly. Cut away and discard the 'choke'; this consists of the central inner leaves with a hairy growth at the base. Allow the artichokes to become completely cold. Serve with the dressing.

Cook's Tip

Choose the avocados carefully, avoiding any that are bruised. The discoloured parts are edible but spoil the appearance of the fruit. It is best to buy slightly under-ripe avocados and leave them in a warm kitchen for 24 hours.

Cook's Tip

The way to test if an artichoke is ready is to lift one out of the water and pull off an outer leaf; it should come away easily and if the inner base of the leaf is tender, the artichoke is ready.

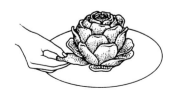

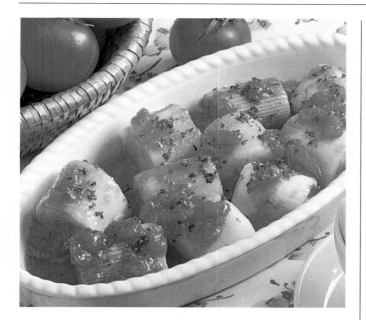

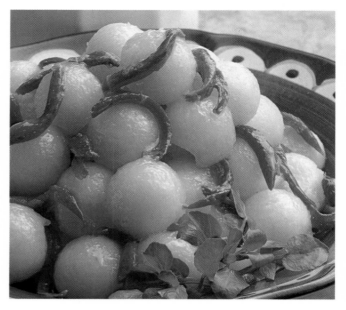

27 | Leeks à la Grecque

Preparation time
10 minutes,
plus cooling

Cooking time
25 minutes

Serves 4

Calories
63 per portion

You will need
350 g/12 oz leeks
juice of ½ lemon
1 tablespoon oil
1 tablespoon water
1 garlic clove, crushed
3 tomatoes, peeled and chopped
salt and pepper
chopped parsley, to garnish

Remove the outer leaves from the leeks and cut into 2.5 cm/1 inch lengths. Wash thoroughly. Place in a pan with the remaining ingredients, adding salt and pepper to taste.

Heat gently to simmering point, then simmer for 20 minutes. Leave to cool in the liquid for about 45 minutes, then arrange in a serving dish and garnish with parsley.

28 | Melon and Anchovy Salad

Preparation time
15 minutes, plus
chilling

Serves 4

Calories
27 per portion

You will need
1 medium melon
1 x 50-g/2-oz can anchovy fillets
juice of 1 lemon
juice of 1 orange
watercress sprigs, to garnish

Halve the melon and discard the seeds. Scoop the flesh into a serving dish, using a melon baller. Alternatively, cut into small cubes.

Drain the anchovy fillets, reserving 1 tablespoon of the oil. Cut the anchovies into short slivers and add to the melon.

Mix the lemon and orange juice with the reserved anchovy oil and pour over the salad. Chill for about an hour before serving, garnished with watercress sprigs.

Cook's Tip

Many people still think of leeks as a vegetable to be served hot in the winter. Young leeks are delicious served as a cold starter. You can use the outer leaves, well washed, in a vegetable stock.

Cook's Tip

Honeydew melons are available all the year round. Check that it is ripe by pressing the stalk end lightly; it should give a little. A ripe melon has a distinctive scent that experts recognize immediately.

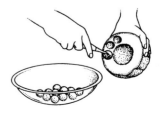

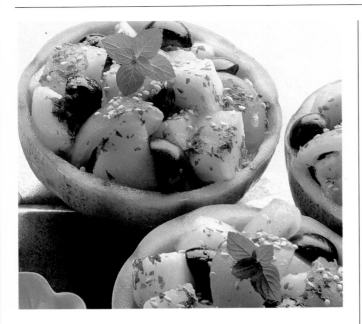

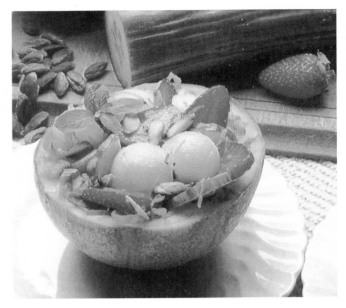

29 | Melon, Tomato and Grape Vinaigrette

Preparation time
20 minutes

Serves 4

Calories
108 per portion

You will need
2 small Ogen melons
4 tomatoes, peeled, quartered and
　seeded
175 g/6 oz black grapes, halved
　and seeded
1 tablespoon sesame seeds,
　roasted
4 mint sprigs, to garnish

For the dressing
2 teaspoons clear honey
5 teaspoons cider vinegar
4 teaspoons oil
1 teaspoon chopped mint
salt and pepper

To make the dressing, put all the ingredients in a screw-topped jar and shake well.

Cut the melons in half and discard the seeds. Scoop the flesh into balls, using a melon baller, or cut into cubes; reserve the shells. Place the melon in a bowl with the tomatoes and grapes. Pour over the dressing.

Toss well, then spoon the mixture into the melon shells. Sprinkle with sesame seeds and garnish with the mint sprigs.

30 | Minted Melon Basket

Preparation time
15 minutes, plus
chilling

Serves 4

Calories
41 per portion

You will need
2 small round melons
75 g/3 oz strawberries or
　raspberries
a few cucumber slices
2 teaspoons chopped mint
1-2 tablespoons fresh orange juice

For the garnish
mint leaves
grated orange rind, finely chopped
　pistachio nuts or toasted
　almonds

Halve the melons and discard the seeds. Scoop the flesh into a bowl, using a melon baller. Mix with the strawberries or raspberries and add a few cucumber slices and the chopped mint. Moisten with the orange juice and spoon the mixture back into the melon shells. Chill for 2 hours.

Top with mint leaves and a sprinkling of grated orange rind, finely chopped pistachio nuts or toasted almonds.

Cook's Tip

Sesame seeds are available in large supermarkets and health food shops. To roast, sprinkle the seeds over a baking sheet and cook in a moderate oven (180°C, 350°F, gas 4) for 15 minutes. Stir them frequently to prevent them blackening.

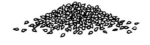

Cook's Tip

The amount of orange juice depends on how juicy the melons are. When soft fruit is out of season, use skinless segments of orange instead of the strawberries or raspberries. The mixture will just take longer to prepare!

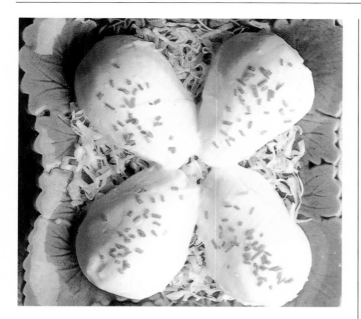

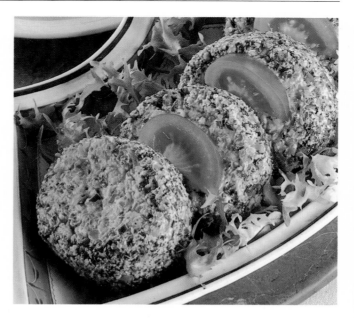

31 | Pears with Curd Cheese

Preparation time
15 minutes, plus
chilling

Serves 4

Calories
151 per portion

You will need
50 g/2 oz Stilton cheese
150 ml/ ¼ pint natural low-fat
    yogurt
100 g/4 oz curd cheese
salt and pepper
2 ripe dessert pears

For the garnish
shredded lettuce leaves
1 tablespoon chopped chives

Mash the Stilton cheese with 1 tablespoon of the yogurt and set aside.

Place the curd cheese in a bowl and beat in the remaining yogurt, and salt and pepper to taste.

Peel, halve and core the pears. Divide the Stilton filling between each cavity.

Arrange the lettuce on a serving dish and place the pears, cut side down, on top. Spoon over the yogurt and curd cheese mixture and sprinkle with the chives. Serve chilled.

32 | Hazelnut and Vegetable Roll

Preparation time
20 minutes, plus
chilling

Serves 4

Calories
223 per portion

You will need
225 g/8 oz low-fat soft cheese
75 g/3 oz toasted hazelnuts,
    chopped
2 celery sticks, finely chopped
1 small green pepper, seeded and
    finely chopped
2 spring onions, finely chopped
1 carrot, finely grated
3 tablespoons chopped parsley
salt
pinch of cayenne pepper
radicchio or endive leaves
2 large tomatoes, thinly sliced

For the coating
3 tablespoons chopped fresh
    parsley
2 tablespoons toasted hazelnuts,
    chopped
2 tablespoons medium oatmeal

Mix together the cheese, nuts, celery, green pepper, onion, carrot and 3 tablespoons parsley. Season with salt and cayenne pepper. Beat the mixture well and shape it into a roll about 7.5 cm/3 inches in diameter. Wrap the roll in foil and chill it for 2-3 hours.

Make the coating. Mix together the parsley, nuts and oatmeal. Roll the cheese mixture in the coating until it is evenly covered. Line a serving dish with the salad leaves. Place the roll on them and garnish it with the tomato slices.

Cook's Tip

Chives can be grown successfully in a flower pot on a sunny window-sill if you do not have a garden. The easiest way to chop them is to hold a few firmly in one hand and snip off tiny pieces with a pair of sharp scissors.

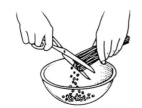

Cook's Tip

If you would like to serve this roll for lunch, prepare it the previous day and chill it overnight. You will then only have to roll the cheese mixture in the coating just before serving it.

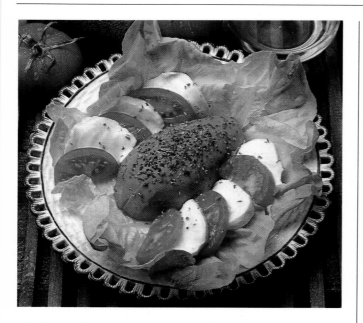

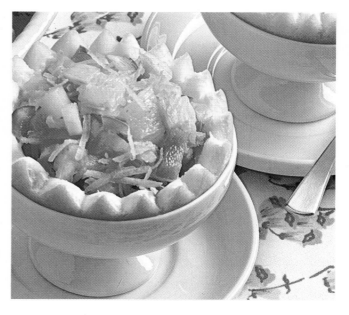

33 | *Avocado Salad*

Preparation time
15 minutes

Serves 4

Calories
268 per portion

You will need
4 large lettuce leaves
3 tablespoons oil
4 teaspoons white wine vinegar or
    lemon juice
salt and pepper
2 avocados
4 tomatoes, peeled and sliced
75 g/3 oz curd cheese
1 teaspoon finely chopped fresh
    marjoram

Arrange the lettuce on four individual serving plates. Blend the oil, vinegar or lemon juice and a little seasoning together.

Halve the avocados, peel and remove the stones. Place on the lettuce leaves, cut side down; slice carefully. Arrange the tomato and cheese slices on the lettuce. Top with the dressing and the marjoram. Serve immediately.

34 | *Tangy Grapefruit*

Preparation time
15 minutes, plus
chilling

Serves 4

Calories
25 per portion

You will need
2 large grapefruit, halved
½ green pepper, seeded and
    chopped
1 carrot, grated
2.5 cm/1 inch piece of cucumber,
    diced
freshly ground black pepper

Loosen the grapefruit from the skin and remove, leaving the empty half grapefruit shells intact. Scallop the edges of the shells, if wished.

Remove the pith and discard. Chop the fruit and place in a bowl with the juice. Add the remaining ingredients, with pepper to taste, and mix well. Cover the bowl with cling film and chill for at least 1 hour.

Just before serving, pile the mixture into the prepared grapefruit shells.

Cook's Tip

If fresh marjoram is not available, replace with ½ teaspoonful of dried oregano. The inclusion of curd cheese in this recipe adds protein, making it a good choice for a light meal as well as a starter.

Cook's Tip

If the grapefruit shells tend to roll around in the dish, carefully remove a thin slice from the base of each half with a sharp knife before filling them. It will then be much easier to eat the fruit.

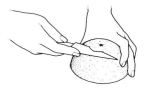

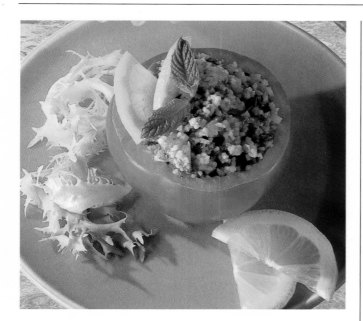

35 | Burghul Tomato Cases

Preparation time
25 minutes, plus
soaking and standing

Serves 4

Calories
149 per portion

You will need
50 g/2 oz fine cracked wheat
  (burghul)
¼ teaspoon salt
2 tablespoons lemon juice
8 large tomatoes
2 spring onions, finely chopped
8 tablespoons chopped fresh
  coriander or parsley
2 tablespoons chopped fresh mint
2 tablespoons olive oil
freshly ground black pepper

For the garnish
salad leaves or vine leaves
mint sprigs
thin slices of lemon

Soak the cracked wheat in water for 15 minutes. Drain it, tip it into a clean tea towel and wring tightly to remove the excess moisture. Turn the cracked wheat into a bowl, sprinkle with salt and lemon juice and set aside for 1 hour.

Cut the tops from the tomatoes. Using a teaspoon or vegetable baller, scoop out the flesh and seeds and chop. Dry the tomato cases with absorbent kitchen paper. Stir the chopped tomato, spring onion, herbs and oil into the cracked wheat and season it with pepper.

Spoon the salad into the tomato cases. Place the tomato cases on a serving dish lined with salad leaves or vine leaves and garnish with mint springs and lemon.

Cook's Tip

If necessary, cut a very thin slice from the base of each tomato so that they stand evenly on the serving dish. Choose tomatoes that are ripe but still quite firm for ease of handling.

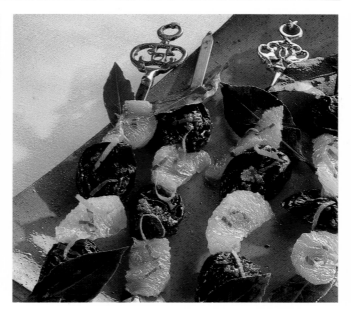

36 | Sunshine Fruit Kebabs

Preparation time
15 minutes, plus
marinating

Cooking time
6-7 minutes

Serves 4

Calories
173 per portion

You will need
2 oranges
2 small grapefruit, peeled and
  segmented
8 pre-soaked prunes, stoned
4 tablespoons vegetable oil
1 tablespoon red wine vinegar
freshly ground black pepper
2 tablespoons chopped fresh mint
8 bay leaves

Peel and segment 1 orange. Cut the other orange in half lengthways. Peel and segment one half. Squeeze the juice and grate the rind from the other half. Thread the orange and grapefruit segments and the prunes on to four skewers. Place them on a flat dish.

Mix together the orange juice, orange rind, oil and vinegar, season with pepper and stir in the mint. Pour the dressing over the kebabs and turn them to coat them thoroughly. Set the kebabs aside for at least 1 hour, turning them occasionally if possible.

Place the kebabs under a preheated moderate grill and cook for 6-7 minutes, turning frequently until the fruit is brown. Thread a bay leaf at both ends of each skewer. Serve hot.

Cook's Tip

Kebabs can also be cooked on a barbecue which is a very popular form of entertaining. These fruit kebabs are also perfect for any vegetarian guests. Remember to turn the kebabs frequently so that they brown evenly.

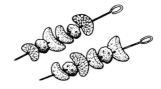

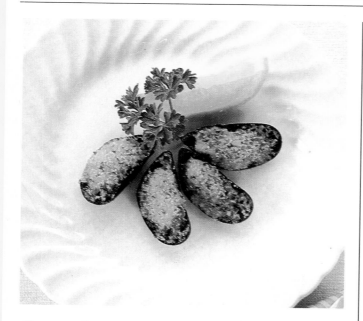

37 | *Stuffed Mussels*

Preparation time
20 minutes

Cooking time
12-14 minutes

Oven temperature
200°C, 400°F, gas 6

Serves 4

Calories
155 per portion

You will need
48 fresh mussels, scrubbed clean
salt
2 lemon slices
2 teaspoons lemon juice
50 g/2 oz soft margarine
1 tablespoon olive oil
3 garlic cloves, crushed
1 shallot, finely chopped
2 tablespoons chopped parsley
3 tablespoons fresh wholemeal
   breadcrumbs

For the garnish
parsley sprigs
lemon wedges

Put the mussels in a pan of boiling salted water, add the lemon slices, cover and cook for about 7 minutes, until the mussels have opened. Remove with a slotted spoon, discarding any that have not opened. Remove the empty top shells from the mussels and discard.

Beat the remaining ingredients together and spread the mixture on top of the mussels. Place on a baking sheet and cook in the oven for 5 minutes or until golden.

Arrange on a warmed serving dish and garnish with the parsley and lemon.

38 | *Scallops with Dill and Lime*

Preparation time
10 minutes, plus
chilling

Cooking time
5 minutes

Serves 4

Calories
85 per portion

You will need
juice of 2 limes
350 g/12 oz queens or scallops
salt and pepper
2 tablespoons chopped dill
1 tablespoon chopped mint
¼ cucumber, diced
2 teaspoons sunflower oil

For the garnish
lime slices
mint sprigs

Pour the lime juice into a saucepan, add the queens or scallops, and salt and pepper to taste. Bring to the boil, then simmer for 2-3 minutes, until the shellfish turn white.

Remove from the heat and allow to cool. Add the dill, mint, cucumber and oil and place in a serving dish. Chill for 2 hours to allow the flavours to develop.

Garnish with lime slices and mint sprigs.

Cook's Tip

Maybe because mussels are among the least expensive varieties of shellfish, they tend not to be fully appreciated in the British Isles. If you feel daunted by the amount of preparation needed, buy ready-cleaned mussels which only need rinsing and the beards pulling off.

Cook's Tip

Queens are smaller than scallops and are ideal for starter dishes. Scallops, like oysters, are best when there is an 'R' in the month, so this is a good dish to serve at a spring or autumn dinner party.

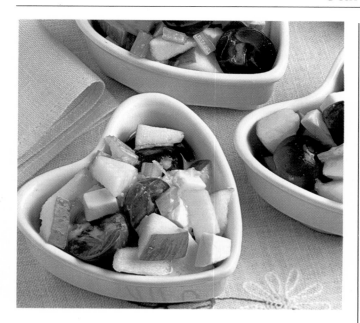

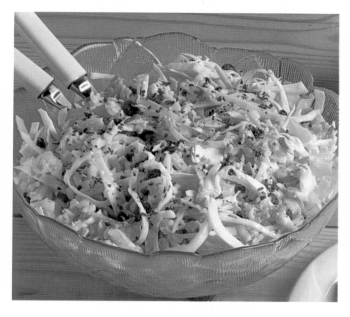

39 | *Cheese and Fruit Cocktail*

Preparation time
20 minutes, plus chilling

Serves 4

Calories
95 per portion

You will need
2 dessert apples
lemon juice
2 celery sticks, chopped
50 g/2 oz Edam cheese, diced
100 g/4 oz grapes, halved and seeded
½ lettuce, shredded
grated rind and juice of 1 orange
2 tablespoons natural low-fat yogurt

Chop the apples and put in a bowl and sprinkle with lemon juice. Add the celery, cheese and grapes and mix together. Arrange a little shredded lettuce in the base of four dishes. Pile the cheese and fruit mixture on top.

Mix the orange rind, juice and yogurt together, then pour a little over each cocktail. Serve chilled.

40 | *Cheese Slaw*

Preparation time
20 minutes

Serves 4

Calories
275 per portion

You will need
250 g/9 oz white cabbage, finely shredded
1 celery stick, chopped
2 carrots, grated
25 g/1 oz raisins
1 dessert apple
2 teaspoons lemon juice
175 g/6 oz Gouda cheese, coarsely grated
150 ml/¼ pint natural low-fat yogurt
salt and pepper
chopped parsley, to garnish

Place the cabbage, celery, carrot and raisins in a large bowl. Grate the apple and toss in the lemon juice. Add to the bowl with the cheese and mix well.

Season the yogurt with salt and pepper to taste, then stir into the salad. Pile on to a serving dish and garnish with chopped parsley.

Cook's Tip

Always wash fresh fruit thoroughly in cold water. This is particularly necessary when using unpeeled fruit such as apples and grapes. A crisp variety of dessert apple will give a pleasant contrasting texture to the cheese.

Cook's Tip

A good dish to serve in the winter when green salad leaves are expensive. The easiest way to prepare the white cabbage is to cut it into thin slices with a serrated bread knife, then chop the shreds to a suitable size.

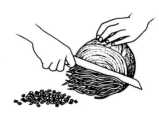

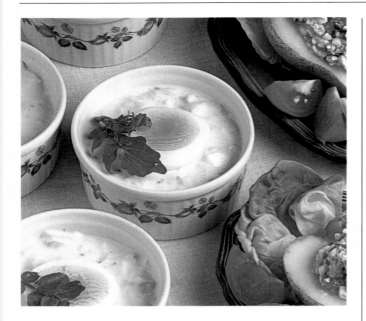

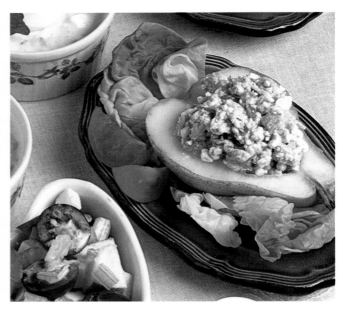

41 | Haddock and Egg Mousse

Preparation time
15 minutes, plus setting

Cooking time
10 minutes

Serves 4

Calories
109 per portion

You will need
175 g/6 oz smoked haddock
1 hard-boiled egg, chopped
200 ml/7 fl oz natural low-fat yogurt
1 teaspoon powdered gelatine
1 tablespoon water
1 teaspoon lemon juice
salt and pepper

For the garnish
watercress sprigs
hard-boiled egg slices

Poach the haddock in a little water for 6 minutes. Drain, skin and flake the fish. Mix with the egg and yogurt.

Dissolve the gelatine in the lemon juice and water in a small bowl over a pan of simmering water. Cool and fold into the fish mixture with salt and pepper to taste. Spoon into four ramekin dishes and chill for about 2 hours, until set. Garnish with watercress and egg.

42 | Crunchy Stuffed Pears

Preparation time
10 minutes

Serves 4

Calories
117 per portion

You will need
2 dessert pears
lemon juice
100 g/4 oz cottage cheese
25 g/1 oz walnuts, chopped
25 g/1 oz raisins
½ red dessert apple, grated
Worcestershire sauce
salt and pepper
lettuce and tomato, to garnish

Cut the pears in half, remove the core and sprinkle with lemon juice. Place the remaining ingredients in a bowl, adding Worcestershire sauce, salt and pepper to taste; mix well.

Pile the mixture into the pear halves, place each one on a lettuce leaf and garnish with lettuce and tomato.

Cook's Tip

If you omit the garnish, you can cover the ramekins with cling film and include them in a picnic basket. They are equally useful as part of a packed lunch accompanied by a tomato salad.

Cook's Tip

If you do not like the taste of their skin, eat these pears with a teaspoon, like a halved avocado. The crunchy cottage cheese filling makes a delicious combination with the texture of the fruit.

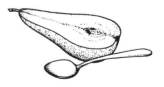

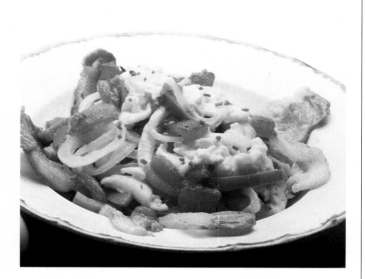

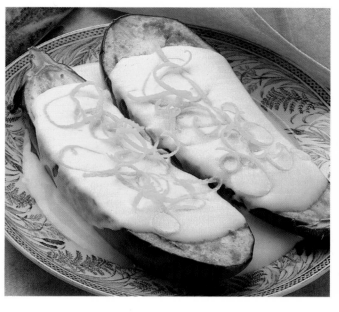

43 | *Pipérade*

Preparation time
15 minutes

Cooking time
15-20 minutes

Serves 4

Calories
384 per portion

You will need
1 tablespoon olive oil
1 large onion, sliced
4 green peppers, seeded and
    sliced
750 g/1½ lb tomatoes, peeled and
    chopped
1 garlic clove, crushed
salt and pepper
1 tablespoon chopped basil
4 small gammon rashers, trimmed
4 eggs, beaten

Heat the oil in a frying pan. Add the onion and fry gently until soft. Add the peppers, tomatoes, garlic, and salt and pepper to taste. Cook until the tomatoes are pulpy. Add the basil.

Meanwhile, cook the gammon under a preheated moderate grill until tender, turning once. Place on a warmed serving dish and keep warm.

Add the eggs to the frying pan and stir until just scrambled. Remove from the heat and pile on top of the gammon. Serve immediately.

44 | *Turkish Aubergines*

Preparation time
10 minutes

Cooking time
25-30 minutes

Oven temperature
200°C, 400°F, gas 6

Serves 4

Calories
167 per portion

You will need
2 aubergines
salt
ground mace
2 teaspoons olive oil
shredded rind of 1 orange, to
    garnish

For the dressing
300 ml/½ pint natural low-fat
    yogurt
2 teaspoons olive oil
2 teaspoons fresh orange juice
pinch of ground mace
salt and pepper

Halve the aubergines lengthways and sprinkle with a little salt and mace.

Cut four pieces of foil each large enough to contain an aubergine half. Lightly brush each aubergine half with oil and wrap in the foil. Bake for 25-30 minutes, or until tender.

Meanwhile, to make the dressing, mix together the yogurt, olive oil, orange juice, mace and salt and pepper.

Unwrap the aubergines and place on a serving dish. Pour the dressing over the hot aubergine halves, sprinkle with orange rind and serve immediately.

Cook's Tip

As gammon tends to be rather salty, use the minimum of salt to season the vegetable mixture. Choose a light main course to follow this substantial starter or perhaps just a fruit dessert.

Cook's Tip

For a sharper-tasting dressing, substitute lemon juice for the orange juice. Use finely chopped mint instead of orange rind as a garnish. The cooking time depends upon the size of the aubergines.

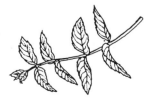

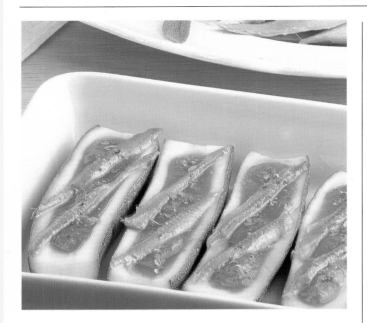

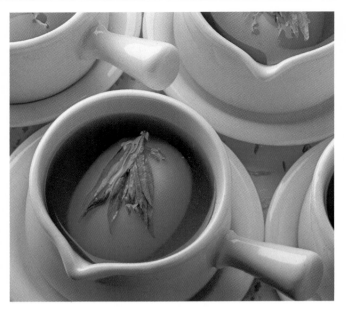

45 | *Zucchini al Forno*

Preparation time
15 minutes, plus
cooling

Cooking time
55 minutes

Oven temperature
200°C, 400°F, gas 6

Serves 4

Calories
61 per portion

You will need
5 large or 10 small courgettes,
   trimmed
salt and freshly ground black
   pepper
1 teaspoon oil
1 garlic clove, finely chopped
1 x 500-g/1¼-lb can tomatoes
1 x 50-g/2-oz can anchovies,
   drained
1 teaspoon chopped marjoram
   (fresh or dried)

Slice the courgettes in half lengthways, and scoop out the seeds and pulp with a teaspoon. Sprinkle the inside of each courgette with salt and leave to drain upside down on absorbent kitchen paper.

Heat the oil in a saucepan and lightly fry the garlic. Rub the tomatoes through a sieve to remove the seeds and add the pulp to the pan. Bring to the boil and cook vigorously until reduced by half. Remove from the heat and stir in one chopped anchovy fillet and half the marjoram.

Wipe the insides of the courgettes with absorbent kitchen paper to remove the salt and set them in a large baking dish; fill each one with the tomato sauce and arrange anchovy fillets on top. Grind over plenty of black pepper and bake for about 40 minutes. Allow to cool before serving, sprinkled with the remaining marjoram.

46 | *Oeufs en Gelée à l'Estragon*

Preparation time
15 minutes, plus
infusing and chilling

Cooking time
8-9 minutes

Serves 4

Calories
120 per portion

You will need
4 eggs
1 x 400-g/14-oz can consommé
6 tarragon sprigs
2 slices Parma ham, trimmed and
   halved
4 tarragon leaves, to garnish

Boil the eggs for 5-6 minutes. Remove from the saucepan, cool in cold water, then shell carefully.

Put the consommé in a saucepan with the tarragon sprigs; heat gently to simmering point. Remove from the heat and leave to infuse for 15 minutes, then discard the tarragon.

Wrap a piece of ham around each egg. Place the eggs in individual ramekin dishes. Spoon over the consommé and float a tarragon leaf on top. Chill until set.

Cook's Tip

**This Italian way of cooking
courgettes is great for
entertaining. It can be
prepared in advance, covered
with cling film and kept in the
refrigerator until needed.
Sprinkle with marjoram at the
last moment.**

Cook's Tip

**The classic version of this
French dish is made with
home-made jellied
consommé. A good quality
brand of canned consommé
makes a very acceptable
substitute. Fresh tarragon is
available in supermarkets.**

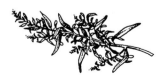

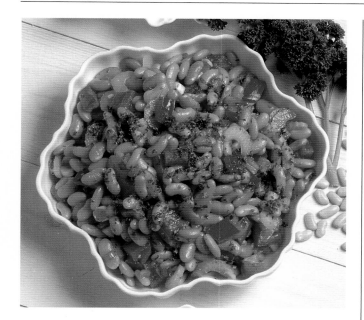

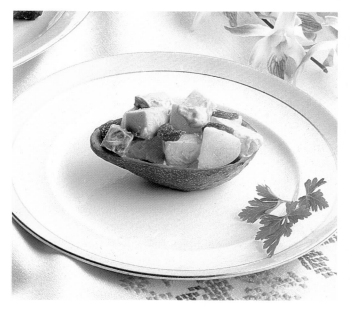

47 | *Flageolets Vinaigrette*

Preparation time
20 minutes, plus soaking overnight and cooling

Cooking time
1 hour 10 minutes

Serves 4

Calories
285 per portion

You will need
250 g/9 oz flageolet beans, soaked overnight
salt
3 tablespoons light French dressing (see Recipe 181)
1 red pepper, seeded and chopped
4 spring onions, chopped
1 tablespoon chopped mixed herbs
2 celery sticks, sliced

Drain the beans, place in a pan and cover with cold water. Bring to the boil and boil rapidly for 10 minutes. Cover and simmer for about 1 hour until tender, adding a little salt towards the end of the cooking. Drain thoroughly and place in a bowl.

Pour over the dressing while still warm and mix well. Leave to cool, then add the remaining ingredients. Toss thoroughly and transfer to a shallow dish to serve.

48 | *Dutch Avocado*

Preparation time
20 minutes

Serves 2

Calories
194 per portion

You will need
1 small avocado
2 tablespoons lemon juice
1 eating apple
25 g/1 oz sultanas
1 teaspoon mild curry powder
2 tablespoons natural low-fat yogurt
salt and pepper

Halve the avocado and remove the stone. Score the flesh into small squares with a sharp pointed knife, cutting through almost to the skin. Scoop the flesh into a bowl and sprinkle with 1½ teaspoons of the lemon juice.

Peel and core the apple and cut into cubes the same size as the avocado. Soak the sultanas in the remaining lemon juice for 5 minutes. Combine the avocado, apple and sultanas.

Mix the curry powder with the yogurt and combine with the avocado mixture. Season with salt and pepper and pile into the avocado skins. Serve immediately.

Cook's Tip

Pulses such as flageolet beans should play an important part in a calorie-controlled diet. They are a rich source of vegetable fibre which provides the essential roughage needed to keep the digestive system healthy.

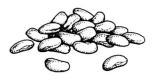

Cook's Tip

If you want to prepare the avocado in advance, cover each filled half tightly with cling film and put in the refrigerator to chill. The lemon juice will help to prevent the avocado flesh from discolouring.

Fish

Many of us grew up with the impression that fish meant fish and chips, with limp white fish deep-fried in greasy batter. Choose instead from the vast selection of fish and seafood which is readily available today. This chapter shows some imaginative ways of preparing this very nutritious, high-protein food. Some of the recipes are primarily for entertaining while others make economical family meals. They include tempting combinations of fish and vegetables such as Seabass Baked with Mangetout, as well as spicy dishes with an Oriental influence like Prawns in Ginger Sauce or Tandoori Sole.

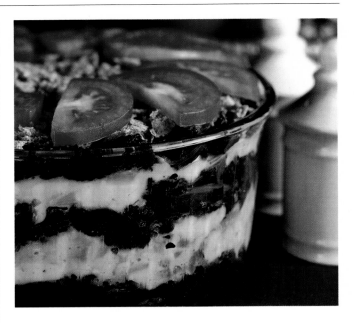

49 | Plaice with Cucumber

Preparation time
15 minutes

Cooking time
5 minutes

Serves 4

Calories
152 per portion

You will need
4 plaice fillets, about 65 g/2 ½ oz each
25 g/1 oz margarine, melted
pepper
1 tablespoon oil
2 spring onions, chopped, including green part
50 g/2 oz mushrooms, thinly sliced
½ cucumber, quartered lengthways, then thinly sliced
juice of 1 lemon
lemon wedges, to garnish

Lay the fish in a lightly oiled grill pan, brush with the melted margarine and season with pepper. Cook under a preheated moderate grill for 3-4 minutes, turning the fish once.

Heat the oil in a frying pan, add the spring onions and fry for 30 seconds, stirring, without browning. Add the mushrooms and stir-fry for 1 minute. Add the cucumber and lemon juice and heat through.

Arrange the fish on warmed serving plates and garnish with the lemon wedges. Serve with the mushroom mixture and grilled tomatoes.

50 | Haddock and Spinach Layer

Preparation time
15 minutes

Cooking time
35-40 minutes

Oven temperature
180°C, 350°F, gas 4

Serves 4

Calories
256 per portion

You will need
500 g/1¼ lb haddock fillets
150 ml/¼ pint skimmed milk
1 bay leaf
salt and pepper
1 hard-boiled egg, chopped
500 g/1¼ lb frozen leaf spinach
2 crispbreads, crushed
1 tomato, sliced, to garnish

For the sauce
about 150 ml/¼ pint skimmed milk
25 g/1 oz margarine
1 onion, chopped
25 g/1oz plain flour
grated nutmeg

Place the haddock in a pan. Add the milk, bay leaf, salt and pepper to taste, then poach for about 10 minutes until the fish is tender. Drain, reserving the liquor. Flake the haddock and mix with the egg.

Cook the spinach as directed on the packet and drain.

Make the fish liquor up to 300 ml/½ pint with extra milk. Melt the margarine in a pan and fry the onion until soft. Stir in the flour and cook for 1 minute. Gradually blend in the milk, then bring to the boil, stirring continuously. Cook, stirring, for a further 1 minute. Stir in the fish mixture; mix well. Layer the spinach and fish mixture in a greased 1.2 litre/2 pint ovenproof dish, finishing with the spinach. Sprinkle with the crispbreads and cook in the oven for 20-25 minutes. Garnish with the tomato.

Cook's Tip

If possible, buy whole plaice and do the filleting yourself. It will take a little time but you will have the trimmings to make stock and your fish will stay fresher as it loses some of its flavour when skinned and filleted.

Cook's Tip

Try to crush the crispbreads quite finely so that they can be sprinkled easily over the spinach. To prevent them flying all over the kitchen, cover the crispbreads with greaseproof paper and press gently with a rolling pin.

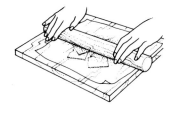

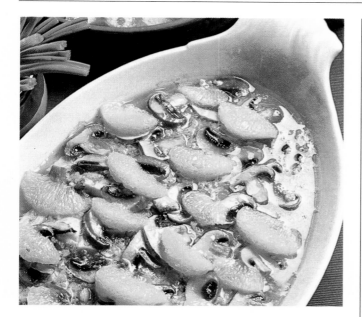

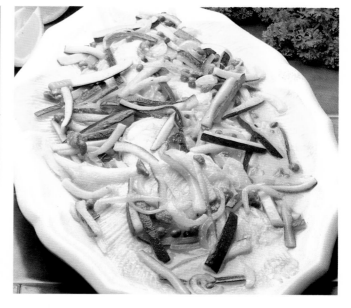

51 | *Haddock with Grapefruit and Mushrooms*

Preparation time
20 minutes

Cooking time
30 minutes

Oven temperature
180°C, 350°F, gas 4

Serves 4

Calories
226 per portion

You will need
4 haddock fillets, skinned, about
175 g/6 oz each
40 g/1½ oz butter or margarine
3 spring onions, chopped
salt and pepper
2 grapefruit
100 g/4 oz mushrooms, sliced

Arrange the haddock fillets in a lightly greased casserole. Mash the butter or margarine with the spring onions and salt and pepper to taste. Grate the rind from the grapefruit and beat into the butter or margarine. Spread this over the haddock fillets. Cover with the mushrooms.

Squeeze the juice from one grapefruit and peel and segment the other. Pour the grapefruit juice over the mushrooms and place the grapefruit segments on top.

Cover and cook in the oven for about 30 minutes, or until the fish is cooked.

52 | *Skate with Courgettes*

Preparation time
20 minutes

Cooking time
20-25 minutes

Oven temperature
200°C, 400°F, gas 6

Serves 4

Calories
400 per portion

You will need
1 ½ teaspoons oil
4 skate wings, rinsed
1-2 tablespoons lemon juice
salt and pepper
lemon slices, to garnish

For the topping
4 courgettes, trimmed
2 tablespoons oil
1 onion, thinly sliced
1 x 50-g/2-oz can anchovy fillets,
drained and chopped
1 tablespoon capers

Put a large sheet of foil on a flat baking sheet. Brush with half the oil. Lay the skate wings side by side on the foil. Sprinkle with the lemon juice and season to taste. Brush a second sheet of foil with the remaining oil and lay over the fish. Press the edges of the two sheets of foil together. Bake in the oven for 20-25 minutes.

Meanwhile, to make the topping, cut the unpeeled courgettes into thick matchstick pieces. Heat the oil in a frying pan, cook the onion until soft, then add the courgettes and continue cooking for 5 minutes. Turn the courgettes once or twice; they should retain a fairly firm texture when cooked. Add the anchovies, capers and a little pepper and heat for 1-2 minutes.

Arrange the skate on a warmed dish, pour any juices left from baking over the fish, then spoon the courgette mixture on top. Garnish with the lemon slices.

Cook's Tip

You will need a sharp knife to peel the grapefruit neatly. Remove the skin in sections, cutting from the stalk end to the base. Cut deeply enough to remove all the pith. Using the tip of a pointed knife, ease out the skinless segments.

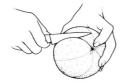

Cook's Tip

The skate will feel sticky because of its gelatinous nature which makes it easy to bone. Rinse well in cold water before cooking. The raw fish smells slightly of ammonia which will disappear when cooked.

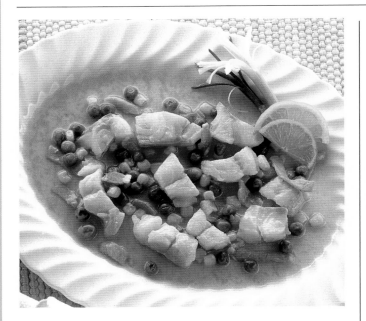

53 | Stir-fried Fish

Preparation time
15 minutes, plus standing

Cooking time
5 minutes

Serves 4

Calories
192 per portion

You will need
500 g/1¼ lb cod fillet, skinned
1 teaspoon salt
1 tablespoon oil
2 rindless rashers back bacon, shredded
50 g/2 oz frozen peas, cooked
50 g/2 oz frozen sweetcorn, cooked
6 tablespoons chicken stock or water
2 teaspoons dry sherry
2 teaspoons soy sauce
1 teaspoon sugar
1 teaspoon cornflour, blended with 1 teaspoon water
spring onion flowers to garnish (see Recipe 96)

Cut the cod fillet into 2.5 cm/1 inch wide strips, sprinkle with salt, leave for 15 minutes.

Heat the oil in a frying pan, add the fish and bacon and stir-fry for 3 minutes. Add the remaining ingredients, except the blended cornflour, and bring to the boil. Stir in the blended cornflour and cook for 1 minute.

Garnish the finished dish with the spring onion flowers and serve immediately.

54 | Fish Casserole with Peppers

Preparation time
15 minutes

Cooking time
25-30 minutes

Oven temperature
180°C, 350°F, gas 4

Serves 4-6

Calories
135 per portion

You will need
1 tablespoon oil
3 spring onions, chopped, including green part
1 green pepper, seeded and cut into strips
1 red pepper, seeded and cut into strips
1 x 400-g/14-oz can chopped tomatoes
½ teaspoon sugar
4-6 frozen cod fillets, thawed
juice of 1 lemon
pepper
1 tablespoon chopped parsley

Heat the oil in a flameproof casserole, add the spring onions and fry for about 1 minute, stirring, without browning. Add the peppers and stir-fry for about 3 minutes.

Add the tomatoes, with their juice, and sugar and bring to the boil. Simmer for 5 minutes, then lay the cod on top. Squeeze over the lemon juice, season with pepper and sprinkle with the parsley. Cover and cook in the oven for 15-20 minutes, depending on the thickness of the fillets.

Serve each portion of fish with some of the pepper mixture.

Cook's Tip

Stir-frying requires less fat or oil than other types of frying. As it also reduces the cooking time to the minimum, it is a boon to busy cooks. The food retains its colour and texture.

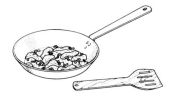

Cook's Tip

Canned chopped tomatoes do cost a little more than the ordinary plum tomatoes. They not only save time but also seem to taste better. Avoid the varieties with herbs if you are adding them to a dish with a well-defined flavour.

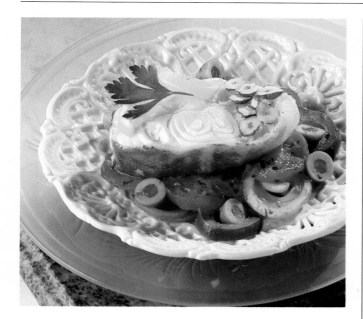

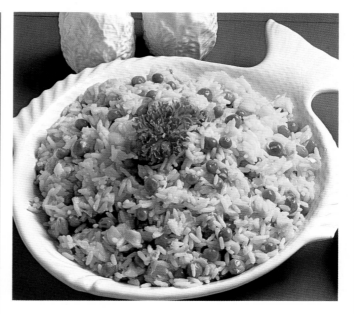

55 | Cod Steaks Riviera

56 | Kedgeree

Preparation time
15 minutes

Cooking time
30 minutes

Serves 4

Calories
199 per portion

You will need
1 large onion, sliced into rings
1 garlic clove, crushed
350 g/12 oz tomatoes, peeled and
    sliced
1 tablespoon tomato purée
1 green pepper, seeded and sliced
    into rings
2 bay leaves
salt and pepper
4 cod steaks, about 175 g/6 oz
    each
1 tablespoon lemon juice
50 g/2 oz stuffed olives, halved
1 tablespoon chopped parsley

For the garnish
25 g/1 oz hazelnuts, chopped
lemon twists
parsley sprigs

Preparation time
15 minutes

Cooking time
25 minutes

Serves 4

Calories
244 per portion

You will need
500 g/1¼ lb smoked haddock
200 ml/7 fl oz skimmed milk
150 g/5 oz long-grain white rice
1 hard-boiled egg, chopped
100 g/4 oz peas, cooked
salt and pepper
parsley sprigs, to garnish

Poach the haddock in the milk for 10 minutes or until tender; drain, reserving the liquor. Flake the fish and remove any skin.

Cook the rice in plenty of boiling salted water for about 12 minutes, or until tender. Drain and rinse thoroughly, then return to the pan. Stir in the fish, eggs, peas and a little of the fish liquor. Season with salt and pepper to taste, then place over a low heat until heated through.

Transfer to a warmed serving dish and garnish with the parsley.

Put the onion, garlic, tomatoes, tomato purée, green pepper rings and bay leaves into a frying pan. Season with salt and pepper, stir well, bring to the boil, cover and simmer over a low heat for 10 minutes. Place the fish steaks on the vegetables, sprinkle on the lemon juice and cover the pan. Simmer for 12-15 minutes, or until the fish is just cooked.

Stir in the olives and parsley and just heat through. Using a fish slice, transfer the fish and vegetable sauce to a warmed serving dish. Discard the bay leaves. Sprinkle on the hazelnuts and garnish with the lemon twists and parsley sprigs.

Cook's Tip

If you wish to use frozen cod steaks, remember to take them out of the freezer in time for them to thaw completely. Pat the fish with absorbent kitchen paper to remove any surplus moisture before cooking.

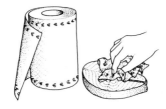

Cook's Tip

This version of the traditional British breakfast dish is a good way to start the day for slimmers. You are much less likely to be tempted to nibble during the morning! It is also a useful supper dish.

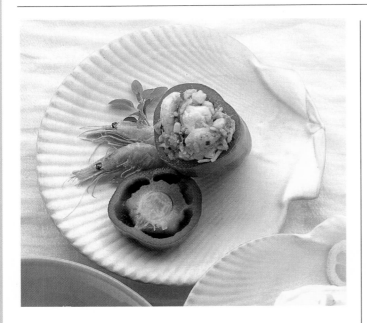

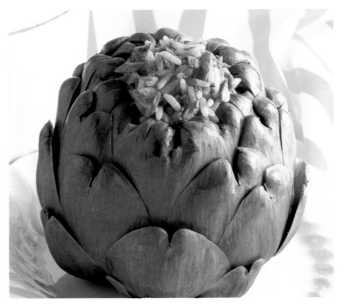

57 | Stuffed Peppers

Preparation time
25 minutes

Cooking time
1¼ hours

Oven temperature
180°C, 350°F, gas 4

Serves 4

Calories
242 per portion

You will need
500 g/1 ¼ lb cod fillets
bouquet garni
½ onion
salt and pepper
1 tablespoon sunflower oil
1 onion, chopped
2 celery sticks, chopped
100 g/4 oz brown rice
1 x 225-g/8-oz can tomatoes
1 bay leaf
1 teaspoon chopped marjoram
100 g/4 oz peeled cooked prawns
4 tablespoons frozen sweetcorn
4 green peppers (see Cook's Tip)
marjoram sprigs
whole cooked prawns

Put the fish in a pan with 300 ml/½ pint boiling water, bouquet garni, onion, and seasoning. Cover and simmer for 10-15 minutes. Remove with a slotted spoon, remove any skin and bones and flake into chunks.

Heat the oil in a frying pan, add the onion and celery and fry for 2 minutes. Add the rice and fry for 3 minutes. Stir in the tomatoes, their juice, bay leaf, marjoram, and seasoning to taste. Add 150 ml/¼ pint cold water, bring to the boil, cover and simmer for 40 minutes, until the rice is tender and the liquid absorbed. Remove from the heat. Stir in the fish, prawns and sweetcorn.

Divide the rice and fish mixture between the peppers. Arrange in an ovenproof dish and replace the reserved tops. Cook in the oven for 15 minutes. Garnish with the marjoram sprigs and prawns.

58 | Tuna-stuffed Globe Artichokes

Preparation time
20 minutes, plus
cooling

Cooking time
25 minutes

Serves 4

Calories
154 per portion

You will need
4 globe artichokes
salt
100 g/4 oz long-grain rice
1 x 350-g/12-oz can tuna fish in
brine
4 tablespoons tomato purée
2 teaspoons chopped fresh basil
or 1 teaspoon dried basil
2 teaspoons chopped fresh
oregano or 1 teaspoon dried
oregano
salt and pepper

Cut off the artichoke stalks. Plunge the heads into boiling salted water. Simmer for about 20 minutes or until the bottom leaves pull away easily. Drain and leave until cold. Remove the hairy chokes from the centre of the artichokes.

Meanwhile, cook the rice in boiling salted water for about 12 minutes. Drain and leave for about 20 minutes, until cold.

Thoroughly drain the brine from the tuna fish and flake it using a fork. Add to the rice together with the tomato purée, herbs and salt and pepper to taste. Fill each globe artichoke with the tuna and rice mixture. Serve with a tomato salad.

Cook's Tip

To prepare the peppers, remove the top from each one and reserve. Remove the core and seeds and trim the base to level. Blanch in a saucepan of boiling water for 2 minutes, drain and plunge into cold water. Drain well.

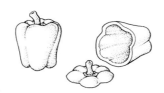

Cook's Tip

Avoid buying tuna fish canned in oil which will add unwanted calories. More rice could be cooked at the same time to be used in another dish the next day; when cold, cover with cling film to prevent it hardening.

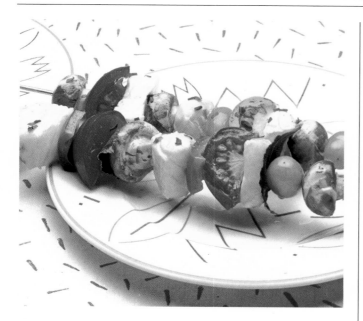

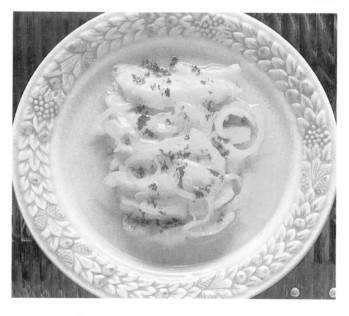

59 | Fish Kebabs

Preparation time
15 minutes

Cooking time
20 minutes

Serves 4

Calories
114 per portion

You will need
1 small green pepper, seeded and
  roughly chopped
450 g/1 lb cod, cut into small
  cubes
4 firm tomatoes, quartered
12 grapes, seeded
8 button mushrooms, trimmed
8 bay leaves
lemon juice
2 teaspoons chopped fresh
  tarragon or 1 teaspoon dried

Put the chopped pepper in a saucepan and simmer in the minimum of water for 10 minutes. Drain.

Thread the fish cubes on to skewers with the tomato quarters, grapes, mushrooms, pieces of pepper and bay leaves. Sprinkle the kebabs with lemon juice and tarragon. Place under a preheated moderate grill for about 10 minutes until the fish is cooked, turning frequently and sprinkling with more lemon juice if necessary.

60 | Cod Sofrito

Preparation time
15 minutes

Cooking time
25-30 minutes

Serves 6

Calories
217 per portion

You will need
1 kg/2 ¼ lb cod fillet, skinned
4 tablespoons olive or corn oil
1 large onion, finely sliced
1 garlic clove, crushed
about 300 ml/½ pint fish stock
3 tablespoons lemon juice
½ teaspoon turmeric
1 x 5-cm/2-inch piece cinnamon
  stick
Maldon or sea salt
freshly ground white pepper
finely chopped parsley, to garnish

Rinse the cod fillet, then cut evenly into thin slices or cubes.

Heat the oil in a large pan, add the onion and cook gently for 10 minutes until softened. Add the garlic and fry gently for another 5 minutes. Add 150 ml/¼ pint of the fish stock, the lemon juice and the turmeric. Bring just to the boil. Add the fish, in one layer if possible, burying the cinnamon stick in the middle. Sprinkle with salt and pepper, then simmer gently for 10-15 minutes, adding 2 tablespoons fish stock every 2-3 minutes and turning the fish once if it is in more than one layer.

Pile on to a serving dish and sprinkle with plenty of chopped parsley.

Cook's Tip

These fish kebabs would be good cooked over a barbecue. Do not then cook meat without cleaning the rack, as the smell of fish can linger, even on metal surfaces. Rub with a cut lemon as a temporary measure.

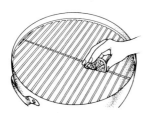

Cook's Tip

When the fish is just cooked, taste the stock and add an extra tablespoonful of lemon juice if necessary. Cod Sofrito is equally good if left until cold, by which time the liquid will have set lightly to give a delicately flavoured jelly.

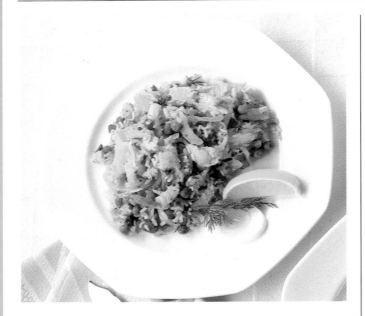

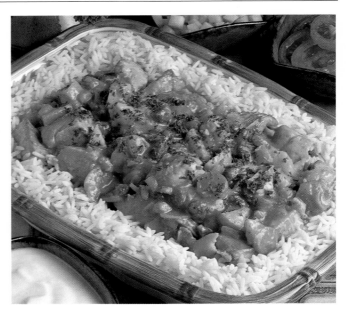

61 | Herb Kedgeree

Preparation time
20 minutes

Cooking time
1 hour 10 minutes

Serves 4

Calories
248 per portion

You will need
350 g/12 oz smoked haddock
25 g/1 oz soft margarine
1 onion, sliced
1 green pepper, seeded and sliced
175 g/6 oz brown long-grain rice,
  washed
grated rind and juice of 1 lemon
2 teaspoons dried mixed herbs
2 bay leaves
25 g/1 oz sultanas
100 g/4 oz peas, cooked
2 tablespoons chopped fresh
  mixed herbs
salt and pepper
1 hard-boiled egg, sliced
lemon wedges
dill sprigs

Poach the smoked haddock in 450 ml/¾ pint water for 10 minutes, then remove fish and reserve stock. Remove the skin and any bones and flake the fish.

Melt the margarine in a large saucepan and sauté the onion and pepper for 2 minutes. Add the rice and cook for a further 2 minutes. Stir in the lemon rind, juice, herbs, bay leaves and reserved stock made up to 900 ml/1½ pints with water. Bring to the boil, cover and simmer for 40 minutes, or until most of the liquid is absorbed. Remove the bay leaves. Stir in the sultanas, peas and fish. Cook for a further 10 minutes, stirring occasionally. Add the fresh herbs and salt and pepper to taste.

Transfer to a warmed serving dish. Garnish with the egg slices, lemon wedges and dill.

Cook's Tip

The choice of fresh herbs can vary the flavour of this kedgeree quite noticeably. Some herbs are better suited to fish dishes than others. Try a mixture of lemon thyme, parsley, marjoram and chives.

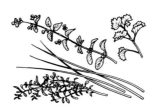

62 | Fish Curry

Preparation time
15 minutes

Cooking time
30-35 minutes

Serves 4

Calories
216 per portion

You will need
25 g/1 oz soft margarine
1 onion, chopped
½ green pepper, seeded and
  chopped
1 carrot, thinly sliced
2-3 teaspoons curry powder
1 tablespoon plain flour
300 ml/½ pint stock
1 teaspoon lemon juice
1 small apple, peeled, cored and
  chopped
1 tablespoon sultanas
500 g/1¼ lb haddock fillets, cut
  into cubes
salt and pepper
chopped parsley, to garnish

Melt the margarine in a pan and fry the onion, pepper, carrot and curry powder for 5 minutes. Stir in the flour and cook for 1 minute. Gradually blend in the stock and lemon juice. Heat, stirring until the sauce thickens. Add the apple, sultanas and haddock, then season to taste with salt and pepper. Cover and simmer for 20-25 minutes.

Transfer to a hot serving dish and garnish with the chopped parsley.

Cook's Tip

The amount of curry powder depends on your personal taste and on the type you are using. This curry should not be too fiery. Serve it with some brown rice which has a nutty texture.

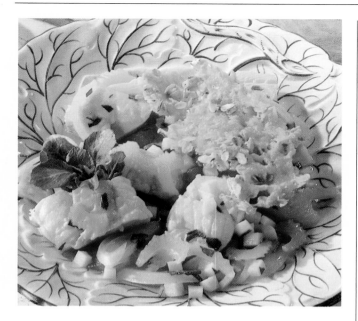

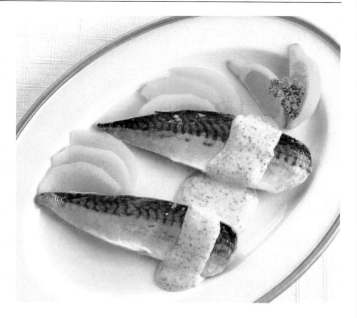

63 | *Haddock and Cider Casserole*

Preparation time
15 minutes

Cooking time
40 minutes

Serves 4

Calories
322 per portion

You will need
1 large onion, sliced
2 celery sticks, thinly sliced
1 garlic clove, chopped
225 g/8 oz tomatoes, peeled and
   sliced
½ bunch watercress, chopped
3 medium potatoes, finely diced
300 ml/½ pint dry cider
2 tablespoons orange juice
strip of thinly pared orange rind
salt and pepper
750 g/1½ lb fresh haddock fillet,
   skinned and cut into 4-cm/
   1½-inch slices
watercress sprigs, to garnish

For the topping
5 tablespoons jumbo oats
40 g/1½ oz low-fat hard cheese,
   grated

Put the onion, celery, garlic and tomatoes into a flame-proof casserole and cook over a low heat for 10 minutes. Add the watercress, potatoes, cider, orange juice and rind. Bring to the boil, cover and simmer for 10 minutes. Season, add the fish, cover and simmer for 10-12 minutes, or until it is just cooked. Discard the rind.

Mix together the oats and cheese and scatter over the dish. Cook under a preheated hot grill for 3 minutes, or until toasty-brown. Garnish with the watercress sprigs and serve hot with chilled low-fat yogurt.

Cook's Tip

Cider has fewer calories than wine and about the same as unsweetened apple juice. If you do not wish to use any alcohol in this casserole, replace the cider with apple juice.

64 | *Baked Mackerel in Cider*

Preparation time
15 minutes

Cooking time
45 minutes

Oven temperature
200°C, 400°F, gas 6;
then 180°C, 350°F,
gas 4

Serves 4

Calories
409 per portion

You will need
1 kg/2 lb cooking apples, peeled,
   cored and thinly sliced
5 tablespoons dry cider
150 g/5 oz, natural low-fat yogurt
5 tablespoons Dijon mustard
salt and pepper
4 mackerel, filleted

For the garnish
lemon slices
parsley sprigs

Spread the apples in a large lightly greased gratin dish.

Heat the cider gently and pour over the apples. Cover with foil and cook in a preheated moderately hot oven for 15 minutes. Lower the temperature to moderate.

Meanwhile, mix the yogurt with the mustard, and salt and pepper.

Arrange the mackerel in the dish and pour over the yogurt mixture. Return to the oven and cook for 30 minutes.

Garnish with lemon slices and parsley before serving.

Cook's Tip

The sharpness of the sauce makes a pleasant contrast to the slightly oily texture of the mackerel. Use one of the grainy Dijon mustards instead of a smooth variety.

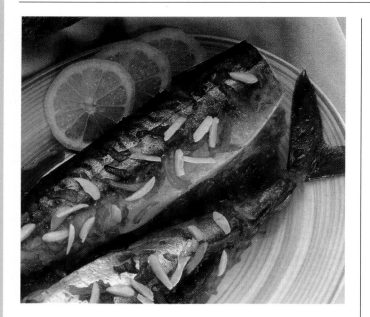

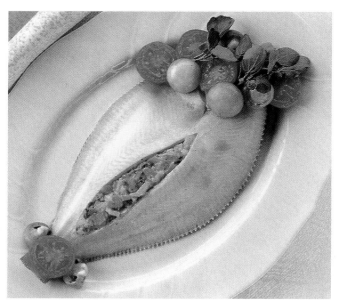

65 | Sweet and Sour Mackerel

Preparation time
20 minutes, plus
marinating

Cooking time
30 minutes

Oven temperature
190°F, 375°F, gas 5

Serves 4

Calories
400 per portion

You will need
4 mackerel

For the marinade
1 small onion, coarsely grated
1 carrot, coarsely grated
2 tablespoons white wine vinegar
  or lemon juice
1 tablespoon brown sugar
1 tablespoon soy sauce
salt and pepper

For the garnish
25 g/1 oz blanched almonds, cut in
  shreds
lemon slices

Remove the heads and intestines from the mackerel and clean them well. Mix the vegetables with the other ingredients for the marinade and pour into a large dish. Place the mackerel in the mixture and leave for 1 hour, turning once or twice.

Lift the fish from the marinade; reserve this. Put the mackerel into an ovenproof dish and bake, uncovered, in the oven for 10 minutes. Pour the marinade over the fish, cover the dish and bake for a further 20 minutes. The vegetables should be slightly firm. Sprinkle the almonds over the fish just before serving. Garnish with lemon slices.

66 | Mushroom-stuffed Plaice

Preparation time
35 minutes

Cooking time
35-40 minutes

Oven temperature
200°C, 400°F, gas 6

Serves 4

Calories
243 per portion

You will need
4 whole plaice, cleaned
1 tablespoon oil
1 onion, finely chopped
1 garlic clove, crushed
75 g/3 oz fresh brown
  breadcrumbs
100 g/4 oz mushrooms, finely
  chopped
1 tomato, peeled and chopped
1 teaspoon chopped marjoram
2 teaspoons chopped parsley
dash of Worcestershire sauce
watercress sprigs, to garnish

Prepare the fish (see Cook's Tip). Heat the oil in a pan, add the onion, garlic and breadcrumbs and fry until the breadcrumbs are crisp. Stir in the remaining ingredients and sauté for 2 minutes. Divide the filling between the prepared pockets in the fish.

Place the fish in a buttered ovenproof dish and cover with foil. Cook in the oven for 20-30 minutes. Garnish with the watercress and serve immediately with grilled tomatoes and mushrooms.

Cook's Tip

Budget-conscious cooks know that mackerel is both nutritious and much less expensive than some other fish. Ask your fishmonger to show you how to remove the intestines from the mackerel and clean them thoroughly.

Cook's Tip

Trim the fish. White side uppermost, make an incision down the backbone. Working from each end of the cut in turn, on one half of the fish, cut two-thirds of the way around to form a pocket. Repeat on the other half.

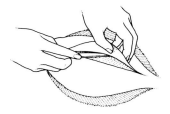

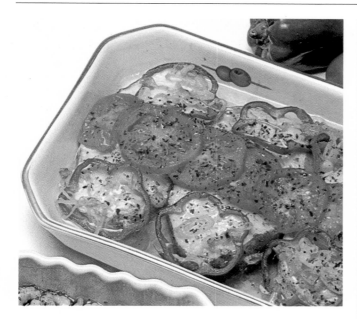
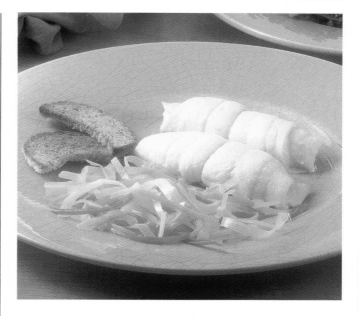

67 | Mediterranean Fish Steaks

Preparation time
15 minutes

Cooking time
55 minutes

Oven temperature
180°C, 350°F, gas 4

Serves 4

Calories
251 per portion

You will need
3 tablespoons olive oil
2 onions, thinly sliced
1 garlic clove, finely chopped
1 green pepper, seeded and sliced in rings
4 large tomatoes, peeled and sliced
2 teaspoons dried basil
salt and pepper
4 white fish steaks, about 175 g/ 6 oz each
2 teaspoons lemon juice
4 tablespoons dry white wine
2 tablespoons water

Heat the oil in a frying pan and fry the onions and garlic until softened. Add the green pepper rings and continue frying for 3 minutes. Remove from the heat and place half the mixture, discarding any oil, in a casserole.

Arrange half the tomato slices on top and sprinkle with half the basil and salt and pepper to taste. Place the fish steaks on top and sprinkle with the lemon juice. Add the remaining tomato slices, basil and onion mixture. Pour in the wine and water. Cover and cook in the oven for about 45 minutes, or until the fish is tender.

Cook's Tip

Any firm, white fish steaks are suitable for this appetizing dish. Ask your fishmonger's advice about the best buy at any particular time of the year and freeze the fish to use later.

68 | Piquant Plaice

Preparation time
20 minutes

Cooking time
13 minutes

Serves 4

Calories
247 per portion

You will need
8 small plaice fillets, skinned, about 65 g/2 ½ oz each
salt and pepper
¼ teaspoon ground ginger
1 small onion, finely chopped
150 ml/¼ pint white wine
150 ml/¼ pint chicken stock
2 green leeks, cleaned and cut into matchstick strips
4 tablespoons low-calorie mayonnaise
4 tablespoons natural low-fat yogurt
1 thin slice fresh root ginger
½ teaspoon mild curry powder
small croûtons, to garnish

Lay the plaice fillets down, skinned sides uppermost, and sprinkle with salt, pepper and ginger. Roll up and secure with wooden cocktail sticks. Scatter the onion in a large frying pan; lay the plaice on top and add the white wine and stock. Cover the pan and simmer gently for about 10 minutes. Meanwhile simmer the strips of leek in boiling water for 3 minutes.

Remove the plaice paupiettes and keep warm. Place the drained strips of leek around the fish.

Mix the mayonnaise with the yogurt. Squeeze the root ginger in a garlic press to extract the juice and add to the mixture with the curry powder and seasonings. Arrange two paupiettes on each plate and garnish with the strips of leek and croûtons. Serve the sauce separately.

Cook's Tip

Most people probably think of croûtons as being small cubes of crisply fried bread used as a soup garnish. These croûtons are made by stamping out crescents from thinly sliced bread and toasting them slowly until crisp.

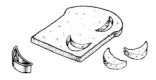

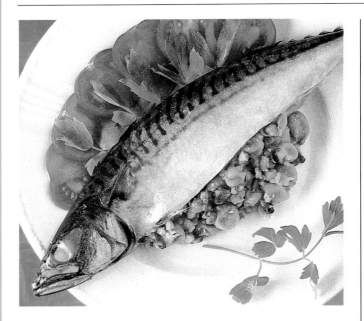

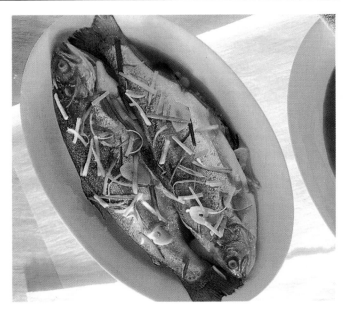

69 | *Mackerel Parcels*

Preparation time
20 minutes

Cooking time
35-45 minutes

Oven temperature
180°C, 350°F, gas 4

Serves 6

Calories
455 per portion

You will need
6 small mackerel, about 275 g/
   10 oz each, cleaned but heads
   and tails left on
Maldon or sea salt
freshly ground white pepper
275 g/10 oz gooseberries, topped
   and tailed
½ teaspoon sugar (optional)
1 teaspoon lemon juice
40 g/1½ oz hazelnuts, finely
   chopped
¼ teaspoon green peppercorns,
   drained if in brine, lightly
   crushed
6 tablespoons dry cider
coriander sprigs, to garnish

Rinse the mackerel, rubbing any traces of blood with a little salt. Rub salt and pepper over the fish; set aside.

To make the stuffing, put the gooseberries into a small pan and add just enough cold water to cover. Bring to the boil, then simmer gently for 10-20 minutes until soft and pulpy and most of the liquid has been absorbed. Taste and add sugar if necessary. Stir in the lemon juice, nuts and peppercorns.

Cut out six pieces of foil, each large enough to enclose the fish with a good edge left to seal the parcels. Stuff each fish, pushing the mixture through the belly cavity. Put each fish on a piece of foil. Sprinkle a tablespoon of cider over each, grind over some white pepper, then seal the parcels tightly. Cook in the oven for 20-25 minutes. Open the parcels and garnish.

Cook's Tip

The fish may be prepared, and the stuffing cooked, up to 3 hours in advance, if covered with cling film and kept cool until you are ready to cook it. On a very hot day, chill the fish and bring to room temperature before stuffing.

70 | *Chinese Steamed Trout*

Preparation time
15 minutes

Cooking time
15 minutes

Serves 4

Calories
340 per portion

You will need
1 teaspoon sesame oil
1 tablespoon light soy sauce
1 tablespoon dry sherry
2 rainbow trout, about 1 kg/2¼ lb
   total weight, cleaned
4 garlic cloves, thinly sliced
6 spring onions, shredded
2 x 2.5 cm/1 inch pieces root
   ginger, shredded
2 tablespoons dry white vermouth
2 tablespoons oil

Mix together the sesame oil, soy sauce and sherry and use to brush the inside and the skin of each fish.

Mix together the garlic, spring onions and ginger and place a quarter of the mixture inside each fish. Put the fish on a heatproof plate, scatter over the remaining garlic mixture and pour over the vermouth and oil. Put the plate in a wok and steam vigorously for 15 minutes, or until the fish is tender.

Arrange the fish on a warmed serving plate, spoon over the juices and serve immediately.

Cook's Tip

A wok is a very useful utensil, both for steaming and stir-frying. Alternatively, you could put the plate on a grill rack in a roasting tin and cover with foil, to make a tent over the fish.

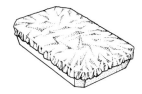

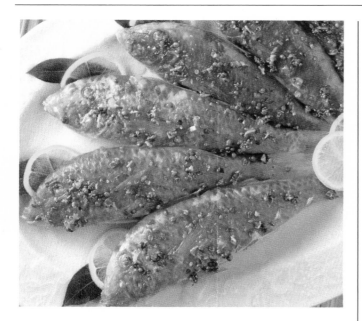

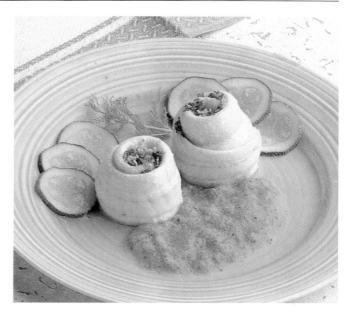

71 | Red Mullet with Coriander Seeds

Preparation time
10 minutes, plus standing

Cooking time
10-12 minutes

Serves 6

Calories
190 per portion

You will need
6 small red mullet, cleaned, livers not removed
3 tablespoons olive oil
2 tablespoons coriander seeds, lightly crushed
3-4 garlic cloves, finely chopped
Maldon or sea salt
freshly ground white pepper

For the garnish
lemon slices
bay leaves

Rinse the mullet quickly and pat dry with absorbent kitchen paper. Brush with 1 tablespoon of the oil and leave for 5 minutes.

Heat the remaining oil in a frying pan, add the coriander seeds and garlic and fry for 2 minutes. Brush the fish with some of this mixture, sprinkle with salt and pepper, and cook under a hot grill for 4-5 minutes. Turn and brush with the remaining oil, then grill for 4-5 minutes until crisp. Garnish and serve immediately.

Cook's Tip

Ideally crush the coriander seeds in a pestle and mortar. Otherwise, try covering the seeds with a piece of greaseproof paper and pressing them with a heavy rolling pin to release their fragrance.

72 | Plaice with Courgette and Lemon Sauce

Preparation time
25 minutes

Cooking time
15 minutes

Serves 4

Calories
169 per portion

You will need
8 small plaice fillets, about 65 g/ 2 ½ oz each, skinned
salt and pepper
finely grated rind of ½ lemon
1 tablespoon finely chopped parsley
300 ml/½ pint skimmed milk

For the sauce
350 g/12 oz courgettes
300 ml/½ pint chicken stock
grated rind of ½ lemon
1 garlic clove, chopped
dill sprigs, to garnish

Spread out the plaice fillets, skinned sides uppermost. Sprinkle with salt and pepper to taste, lemon rind and parsley, and roll each one up, securing with a wooden cocktail stick.

For the sauce, chop the courgettes and cook with the stock, lemon rind and garlic until just tender. Blend the cooked courgettes and their liquid until smooth.

Put the rolled plaice fillets into a shallow pan; add the milk and salt and pepper to taste. Poach the fish gently until it is just tender, about 8-10 minutes, then drain, reserving the liquid. Put on a warmed serving dish.

Heat the courgette purée in a pan with sufficient of the fish cooking liquid to make a fairly thin sauce. Spoon the sauce around the rolled fish fillets and garnish with dill.

Cook's Tip

If you would like to serve a vegetable with the plaice, thinly sliced courgettes are ideal. Poach them gently in chicken stock until they are just tender while the fish is cooking.

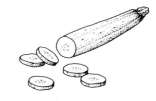

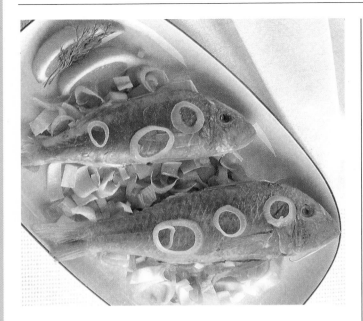

73 | Red Mullet with Chicory

Preparation time
20 minutes

Cooking time
35 minutes

Oven temperature
180°C, 350°F, gas 4

Serves 4

Calories
247 per portion

You will need
350 g/12 oz chicory
salt and pepper
25 g/1 oz unsalted butter
1 small onion, sliced
1 shallot, finely sliced
2 teaspoons lemon juice
salt and pepper
4 small red mullet, cleaned and
   scaled

For the garnish
dill sprigs
lemon wedges

Blanch the chicory in boiling salted water for 5 minutes. Drain, then break off and slice the leaves.

Melt the butter in a pan, stir in the onion, shallot, chicory, lemon juice, and salt and pepper to taste. Cover and cook for 5 minutes.

Spoon into an ovenproof dish. Place the red mullet on top and sprinkle with salt and pepper. Cover with foil and cook in the oven for 20 minutes, or until cooked. Garnish with dill and lemon to serve.

74 | Fish Plaki

Preparation time
15 minutes, plus
cooling

Cooking time
40-45 minutes

Oven temperature
180°C, 350°F, gas 4

Serves 4

Calories
313 per portion

You will need
1 kg/2¼ lb fish fillets, cut into fairly
   thick slices
1 large lemon
3 large onions, thinly sliced
2-3 garlic cloves, finely chopped
¾ teaspoon fresh oregano
3 beefsteak tomatoes, peeled and
   thinly sliced
4 tablespoons finely chopped
   parsley
Maldon or sea salt
freshly ground black pepper
2 tablespoons olive oil
about 300 ml/½ pint water

Arrange the fish in an ovenproof dish. Grate the lemon rind evenly over the fish, then peel off all the pith and cut the flesh into slices. Lay on top of the fish. Add the onion slices, garlic and oregano. Top with the tomatoes and sprinkle over the parsley, salt and plenty of pepper. Mix the oil with the water and pour over the fish. The liquid should just cover all the ingredients, so add a little more water if necessary.

Bake in the oven for 40-45 minutes, or until a fork penetrates the fish very easily. Cool to room temperature (about 25 minutes).

Cook's Tip

Buy the chicory on the same day as you are making the dish if possible. The outer leaves tend to discolour soon and lose their crispness. Sliced fennel can be used instead of chicory.

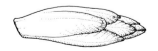

Cook's Tip

John Dory is a delicious fish to choose for this Greek dish. Oregano is the best substitute for the rigani used in Greece. This mixture of dried flowers and leaves of marjoram is not obtainable elsewhere.

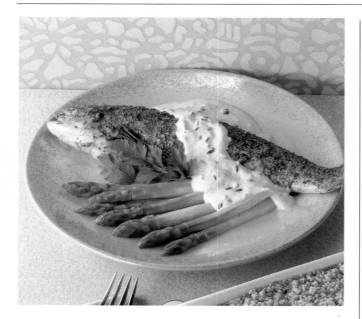

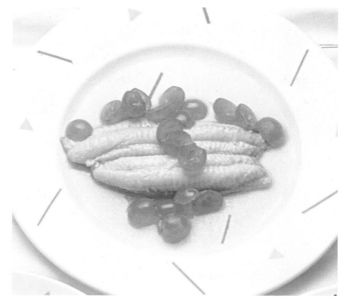

75 | Steamed Trout with Yogurt

Preparation time
20 minutes

Cooking time
10-15 minutes

Serves 4

Calories
275 per portion

You will need
4 trout, gutted and cleaned
4 tablespoons lemon juice
1 tablespoon chopped parsley
1 teaspoon dried thyme
freshly ground black pepper

For the sauce
150 ml/¼ pint natural low-fat
  yogurt
2 tablespoons grated horseradish
  or horseradish sauce
2 tablespoons lemon juice
1 teaspoon white wine vinegar
½ teaspoon dried tarragon
1 teaspoon chopped chives
pinch of cayenne

For the garnish
flat leaf parsley
chives

Put the trout on a large sheet of foil and sprinkle with lemon juice, parsley, thyme and black pepper. Fold into a parcel and place between two large plates. Put these over a pan of boiling water and allow to steam for 10-15 minutes, or until tender. Transfer to a warmed dish.

To make the sauce, put the yogurt, horseradish, lemon juice, vinegar, tarragon, chives and cayenne in a heatproof bowl. Put over a pan of simmering water and stir until hot and creamy. Pour over the trout and serve immediately, garnished with the parsley and chives.

Cook's Tip

Serve boiled new potatoes with the trout. With the creamy yogurt sauce, you will not be tempted to put any butter on the potatoes! Do not add mint to the cooking water as this aromatic herb is very intrusive.

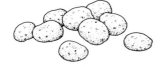

76 | Sole Veronica

Preparation time
15 minutes

Cooking time
20 minutes

Serves 4

Calories
141 per portion

You will need
4 sole fillets, about 100 g/4 oz
  each
250 ml/8 fl oz grape juice
salt and pepper
40 grapes, seeded

Put the sole fillets in a wide shallow pan and pour over the grape juice. Season with salt and pepper. Simmer gently for about 15 minutes until the fish is tender. Add the grapes and cook for a further 5 minutes. Transfer the fish to a warmed serving dish and pour the sauce and grapes over.

Cook's Tip

Both red and white grape juice are available in large supermarkets and health food shops. It is important to read the label carefully to make sure it does not contain any form of sweetening.

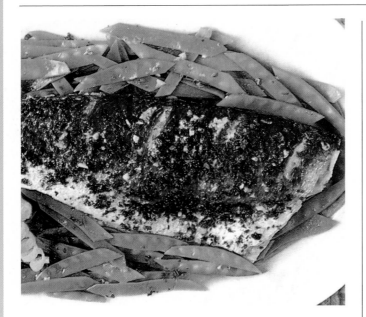

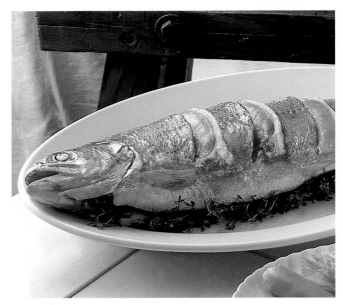

77 | Seabass Baked with Mangetout

Preparation time
5 minutes

Cooking time
45 minutes

Oven temperature
190°C, 375°F, gas 5

Serves 6

Calories
338 per portion

You will need
75 g/3 oz unsalted butter
1.5 kg/3 lb seabass, cleaned, head and tail cut off, fish boned
300 ml/½ pint dry white wine
3-4 garlic cloves, finely chopped
½ teaspoon ground cinnamon
Maldon or sea salt
freshly ground black pepper
6 tablespoons finely chopped parsley
350 g/12 oz mangetout
3-4 tablespoons lemon juice
lemon twists, to garnish

Rub a large ovenproof serving dish with a little of the butter, then place the seabass in it, leaving room on either side to add the mangetout. Cut the remaining butter into small pieces and dot all over the fish, then pour over the wine and sprinkle with the garlic, cinnamon, salt and plenty of pepper, finally covering with the parsley. Lay on a butter paper and cook in the oven for 40 minutes.

Meanwhile blanch the mangetout for 30 seconds in boiling water. Remove the butter paper, put the mangetout around the seabass, spooning a little of the melted butter over them. Sprinkle both the fish and the mangetout with lemon juice and bake for another 5-6 minutes until the mangetout are just cooked but still crunchy and the fish flakes easily when tested with a fork. Garnish and serve immediately.

Cook's Tip

Bream or grey mullet can also be cooked in this way. Although mangetout are available all the year round, they are best value in summer. They only need topping and tailing.

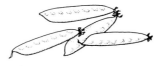

78 | Pike with Beetroot Sauce

Preparation time
15 minutes, plus marinating

Cooking time
45-50 minutes

Oven temperature
190°C, 375°F, gas 5

Serves 6

Calories
238 per portion

You will need
1 pike, weighing about 2 kg/4½ lb, gutted, scaled and cleaned
juice of 1 lemon
salt and pepper
50 g/2 oz rindless back bacon
1 bunch mixed fresh herbs
40 g/1½ oz margarine
250 g/9 oz cooked beetroot
4 tablespoons dry red wine
1 teaspoon sugar
herbs, to garnish

Wash the pike, wipe dry with absorbent kitchen paper and sprinkle inside and out with lemon juice. Leave the fish to marinate for about 10 minutes, then season with salt and pepper to taste.

Make deep cuts on each side of the fish with a sharp knife and fill each cut with a slice of bacon. Stuff the fish with the herbs. Place the fish in a large roasting tin and dot with 25 g/1 oz of the margarine. Cook in the oven for 45-50 minutes.

Meanwhile, to make the sauce, purée the beetroot in a liquidizer with the red wine. Transfer to a small pan and heat gently. Stir in the remaining margarine, sugar, and salt and pepper to taste. Arrange the fish on a warmed platter, garnish with herbs and serve with the sauce.

Cook's Tip

Pike is often caught by anglers in British rivers and lakes but it may be difficult to find in a fishmonger. Another oily fish, such as salmon trout, could be used instead.

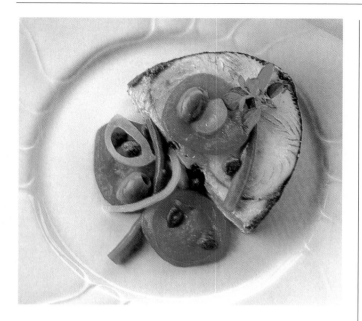

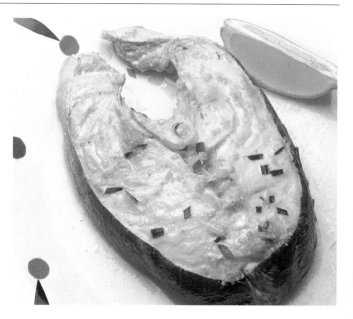

79 | *Swordfish Provençal*

Preparation time
20 minutes, plus marinating

Cooking time
45-50 minutes

Oven temperature
180°C, 350°F, gas 4

Serves 4

Calories
191 per portion

You will need
2 swordfish steaks
1 tablespoon sunflower oil
1 onion, sliced
750 g/1½ lb tomatoes, thickly sliced
250 g/9 oz green beans, cut in half
100 g/4 oz green olives, stoned
2 tablespoons capers
2 teaspoons chopped fresh oregano

For the marinade
150 ml/¼ pint dry white wine
4 tablespoons lemon juice
1 small onion, sliced
1 bay leaf
2 thyme sprigs
2 parsley sprigs
2 rosemary sprigs
2 garlic cloves, crushed
salt and pepper

Cut the swordfish steaks in half, place in a shallow dish and add the marinade ingredients. Chill for 5 hours.

Remove the fish with a slotted spoon; reserve the marinade. Heat the oil in a large pan, add the fish and fry for 5 minutes. Transfer to a casserole. Add the onion, tomatoes, beans, olives, capers, oregano and reserved marinade to the pan and cook, stirring for 5 minutes. Transfer to the casserole and season. Cook in the oven for 35-40 minutes. Discard the bay leaf.

Cook's Tip

So called because of its long sword-like beak, swordfish is a relative newcomer to Britain but an established favourite in Mediterranean countries. It is available in some supermarkets and chain stores.

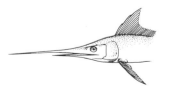

80 | *Halibut with Tarragon*

Preparation time
10 minutes, plus marinating

Cooking time
15-20 minutes

Oven temperature
200°C, 400°F, gas 6

Serves 4

Calories
180 per portion

You will need
4 halibut steaks, about 175 g/6 oz each
grated rind and juice of 2-3 lemons
few tarragon sprigs
salt and pepper

Place the halibut in a large shallow dish. Sprinkle over the lemon rind and juice, tarragon, salt and pepper. Turn the fish to coat with the mixture. Cover and leave to marinate for about 3 hours.

Place each piece of fish on a sheet of foil large enough to enclose it. Spoon over a little of the marinade and wrap up the fish. Cook in the oven for about 15-20 minutes, depending on the thickness of the halibut. Unwrap and serve on a warmed dish.

Cook's Tip

Rinse the halibut steaks in cold water to remove any blood, rubbing with a little salt if necessary. Cod steaks can also be cooked in the same way.

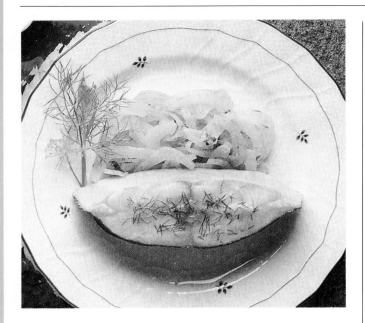

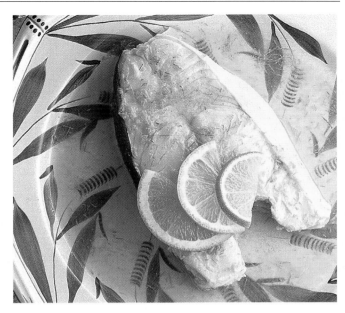

81 | Baked Halibut with Fennel

Preparation time
10 minutes

Cooking time
30-35 minutes

Oven temperature
180°C, 350°F, gas 4

Serves 4

Calories
454 per portion

You will need
6 halibut steaks, about 175 g/6 oz
    each, rinsed
2 large fennel bulbs, finely sliced,
    leaves chopped
40 g/1½ oz butter
2-3 garlic cloves, crushed
100 ml/3½ fl oz dry vermouth
Maldon or sea salt
freshly ground black pepper

Blanch the fennel bulbs in a large pan of boiling water for 2 minutes, then drain thoroughly. Melt the butter, add the fennel bulbs and garlic and cook gently for 10 minutes, or until softened. Spread the fennel, with its butter, over the base of an ovenproof casserole, then add the fish. Pour the vermouth, with a little salt and plenty of pepper, over the fish.

Cook in the oven for 18-25 minutes, until the fish just flakes easily. Serve at once, sprinkled with chopped fennel leaves.

82 | Citrus Halibut Steak

Preparation time
10 minutes, plus
marinating

Cooking time
20 minutes

Oven temperature
180°C, 350°F, gas 4

Serves 2

Calories
100 per portion

You will need
grated rind and juice of 1 orange
grated rind and juice of 1 lemon
grated rind and juice of 1 lime
1 halibut steak, cut in half

For the garnish
2 orange slices
2 lemon slices
2 lime slices

Place 1 tablespoon of each grated rind and all the fruit juices in an ovenproof dish. Add the fish and baste well. Cover and chill for 12 hours, turning the steaks over after 6 hours.

Cover the dish with foil and cook in the oven for 20 minutes. Garnish each portion with an orange, lemon and lime slice.

Cook's Tip

The cooking time varies depending on the thickness of the halibut steaks. Fish should never be overcooked so check if the halibut is ready after 18 minutes.

Cook's Tip

When making this simple dish, remember to prepare it sufficiently early in the day to allow time for it to marinate before cooking. As the steaks should be turned after 6 hours, it is not practical to marinate them overnight!

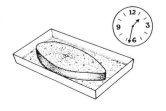

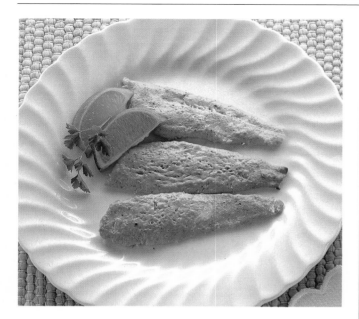

83 | Tandoori Sole

Preparation time
10 minutes, plus
marinating

Cooking time
15 minutes

Oven temperature
180°C, 350°F, gas 4

Serves 4

Calories
117 per portion

You will need
½ teaspoon chilli powder
½ teaspoon turmeric
½ teaspoon ground coriander
½ teaspoon ground cumin
1 teaspoon ground ginger
½ teaspoon garam masala
¼ teaspoon salt
300 ml/½ pint natural low-fat
    yogurt
2 garlic cloves, crushed
4 lemon sole, skinned and filleted

For the garnish
coriander leaves
lime wedges

Mix all the spices together. Add to the yogurt with the
garlic and stir until well mixed. Pour into a large bowl, add
the fish, turn to coat thoroughly and leave to marinate for
1 hour.

Pour boiling water into a roasting pan to come halfway
up the sides. Put a grill rack in the pan and place the mar-
inated fish on the rack. Pour any remaining marinade over
the fish. Cook in the oven for 15 minutes. Garnish with
coriander and lime wedges and serve immediately.

84 | Seabass Baked in Spinach

Preparation time
30 minutes

Cooking time
30 minutes

Oven temperature
200°C, 400°F, gas 6

Serves 4

Calories
400 per portion

You will need
1 seabass, weighing about 750 g/
    1½ lb, cleaned and gutted
250 g/9 oz spinach
2 shallots, chopped
150 ml/¼ pint dry white wine
3 orange slices, quartered, to
    garnish

For the stuffing
50 g/2 oz fresh breadcrumbs
15 g/½ oz butter, melted
2 tablespoons chopped chervil
1 tablespoon chopped tarragon
1 tablespoon chopped basil
1 tablespoon lemon juice
salt and pepper

Mix the stuffing ingredients together, seasoning with
salt and pepper to taste, and use to stuff the fish cavity.

Put the spinach in a colander in a bowl and pour over
boiling water. Drain thoroughly. Wrap the stuffed seabass in the blanched spinach, leaving the head and tail ex-
posed. Sprinkle the shallots over the base of a gratin dish
and place the fish on top. Pour over the wine. Cover with
foil and cook in the oven for 30 minutes.

Transfer to a warmed serving dish and garnish with
quartered orange slices.

Cook's Tip

**Garam masala is an aromatic
mixture of Oriental spices. It is
best to buy it in a shop with a
brisk turnover of seasonings
used in ethnic cooking. The
limes add a characteristic
tang.**

Cook's Tip

**The seabass should be really
fresh. In choosing it you
should look for firmness of
flesh, brightness of eye and
gleaming skin with its
beautiful steel grey and shiny
silver markings.**

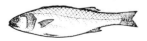

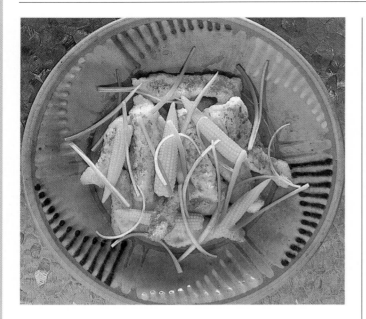

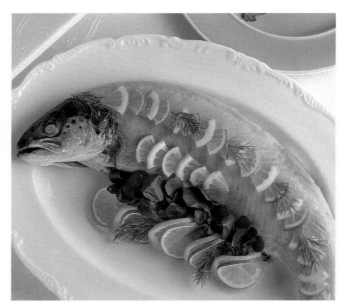

85 | Sole Fillets with Soy and Ginger

Preparation time
15 minutes, plus chilling

Cooking time
10 minutes

Serves 6

Calories
171 per portion

You will need
750 g/1½ sole fillets, skinned
2 egg whites
1 teaspoon cornflour
½ teaspoon Maldon or sea salt
3 tablespoons peanut or grapeseed oil
1 x 5-cm/2-inch piece fresh root ginger, peeled and grated
1 large garlic clove, very finely chopped
3 tablespoons soy sauce
1 tablespoon dry sherry
3 tablespoons fish stock
3 spring onions, cut into matchstick strips

Cut the sole into long thin strips. Beat the egg whites, cornflour and salt until frothy, then pour over the fish, mixing well. Chill for 20 minutes.

Heat the oil in a wok or large frying pan. When nearly smoking, add the fish and stir-fry over a fairly high heat for 2 minutes. Remove from the pan with a slotted spoon, then discard all but 1 tablespoon of the oil. Add the ginger and garlic and stir-fry for 1 minute, then pour in the soy sauce, sherry and fish stock. Bring to the boil quickly, then bubble for 2 minutes. Return the fish to the pan and heat through for 1 minute, stirring constantly. Pile on to a warmed serving dish, sprinkling with the spring onion strips and serve at once.

Cook's Tip

Dip your fingers in cold water and then in salt before you start to skin the sole fillets. It also helps if you first immerse the fish in cold water for 15 minutes. Serve the fillets with baby corn-cobs.

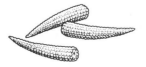

86 | Poached Salmon Trout

Preparation time
35-40 minutes, plus chilling

Cooking time
30 minutes

Oven temperature
150°C, 300°F, gas 2

Serves 6

Calories
341 per portion

You will need
1 salmon trout, weighing about 1 kg/2¼ lb, cleaned and gutted
1 bay leaf
1 lemon, sliced
1 teaspoon salt
12 black peppercorns
300 ml/½ pint dry white wine

For the garnish
½ x 25-g/1-oz packet aspic powder
2 lemons, sliced
2 limes, sliced
small bunch of dill
½ packet of watercress

Line a large roasting pan with foil and brush lightly with the oil. Place the salmon trout on the foil, curving the fish slightly. Place the bay leaf and lemon slices on the fish, then sprinkle with the salt and peppercorns. Pour over the wine. Bring the edges of foil together and seal.

Cook in the oven for 30 minutes. Leave to cool in the pan. Unwrap the fish, remove the skin, leaving some around the head and tail, and place on a serving dish.

Make up the aspic to 300 ml/½ pint according to packet directions. Coat the fish with a thin layer of aspic jelly. Cut most of the lemon and lime slices into quarters and arrange down the centre of the fish with the dill. Brush the lemon and lime slices with a little aspic jelly. Chill in the refrigerator until set (about 2½ hours). Garnish with any remaining lemon and lime slices and watercress.

Cook's Tip

If you do not have a fish kettle, this is the best way of poaching a salmon trout. Allow the coating of aspic jelly to set slightly before adding the lemon and lime slices.

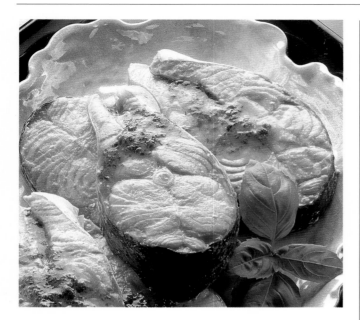

87 | Poached Salmon Steaks with Hot Basil Sauce

Preparation time
15 minutes

Cooking time
25 minutes

Serves 6

Calories
169 per portion

You will need
1 large bunch fresh basil
4 celery sticks, chopped
1 carrot, chopped
1 small courgette, chopped
1 small onion, chopped
6 salmon steaks, about 100 g/4 oz
    each and 2.5 cm/1 inch thick
85 ml/3 fl oz dry white wine
120 ml/4 fl oz water
salt and pepper
1 teaspoon lemon juice
15 g/½ oz unsalted butter

Strip the leaves off half the basil and set aside. Spread all the chopped vegetables over the bottom of a large flameproof dish with a lid, press the salmon steaks into the vegetables and cover them with the remaining basil. Pour over the wine and water and add salt and pepper to taste. Bring to the boil, cover and simmer for about 10 minutes. Transfer the salmon to a warmed serving dish.

    Bring the poaching liquid and vegetables back to the boil and simmer for 5 minutes. Strain into a liquidizer and add the cooked and uncooked basil. Blend to a purée and return to a saucepan. Bring the purée to the boil and reduce by half, until thickened. Remove the pan from the heat, add the lemon juice and stir in the butter. Pour the sauce over the salmon steaks and serve.

Cook's Tip

Make sure that you do not overcook the salmon. It should be opaque and firm when tested with the point of a sharp knife.

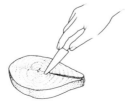

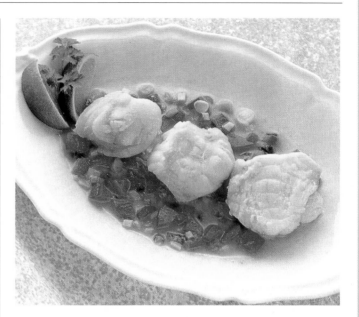

88 | Creamed Coconut Monkfish

Preparation time
20 minutes, plus
infusing

Cooking time
10-15 minutes

Serves 4

Calories
360 per portion

You will need
100 g/4 oz desiccated coconut
300 ml/½ pint boiling water
750 g/1½ lb monkfish
1 tablespoon oil
6 spring onions, chopped
3 green chillies, seeded and
    chopped
1 red pepper, seeded and
    chopped
1 garlic clove, crushed
1 x 5 cm/2 inch piece fresh root
    ginger, chopped
½ teaspoon ground cumin
½ teaspoon ground coriander
1 teaspoon grated lemon rind
1 tablespoon lime juice
1 tablespoon dry sherry
salt and pepper

For the garnish
lime wedges
coriander leaves

Put the coconut in a bowl, pour over the boiling water and leave to infuse for 30 minutes. Strain and reserve the liquid, discarding the coconut.

    Meanwhile, cut the fish into 5 cm/2 inch cubes. Heat the oil in a large pan and stir in the remaining ingredients. Add the fish, pour on the coconut milk and bring to the boil, then simmer for 5 minutes. Transfer to a warmed serving dish and garnish with lime and coriander.

Cook's Tip

In some areas monkfish is known as angler fish. Unfortunately it tends to be rather expensive. It is also delicious when grilled and served cold with an avocado salad.

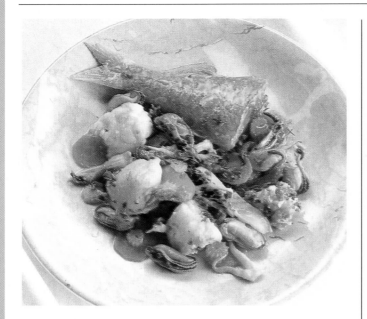

89 | *Fish Casserole*

Preparation time
45 minutes

Cooking time
30-35 minutes

Serves 6

Calories
238 per portion

You will need
12 mussels, cleaned
salt and pepper
1 monkfish, cleaned and filleted
2 squid, cleaned
2 tablespoons oil
2 onions, chopped
2 carrots, thinly sliced
6 celery sticks, sliced
2 garlic cloves, crushed
1 x 400-g/14-oz can tomatoes
2 teaspoons sugar
2 tablespoons lemon juice
2 tablespoons lime juice
2 tablespoons chopped coriander
bouquet garni
150 ml/¼ pint dry cider
few drops Tabasco
4 scallops, cleaned and cut in half
    horizontally
3 small red mullet, cleaned

Put the mussels in a saucepan of boiling salted water and cook for about 7 minutes, until they open; discard any that do not open. Cut the monkfish into 2.5 cm/1 inch chunks. Cut the squid into thin slices; leave the tentacles in small pieces.

Heat the oil in a large saucepan, add the onions, carrots, celery and garlic and sauté for 4 minutes. Add the remaining ingredients, except the fish, with salt and pepper to taste, and bring to the boil. Add all the fish except the mussels, cover and simmer for 15-20 minutes, until the fish is cooked. Discard the bouquet garni. Stir in the mussels and transfer to a warmed serving dish.

Cook's Tip

A wonderful casserole to make if you are lucky enough to have an enterprising fishmonger who can supply all the different types of fish and shellfish. You may have to order the squid in advance.

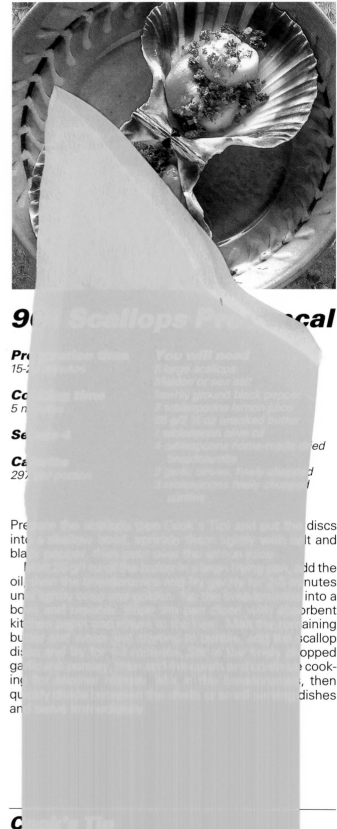

9[0] | *Scallops P[rovençal]*

Pr[eparation time]
15-2[...]

Co[oking time]
5 m[...]

Se[rves 4]

Ca[lories]
29[...]

Pre[...] the scallops (see Cook's Tip) and put [...] discs into [...]lt and bla[...]

[...]dd the oil, [...]nutes un[...] into a bo[...]rbent kit[...]aining bu[...]callop dis[...]opped ga[...] cook ing [...], then qu[...]dishes an[...]

C[ook's Tip]

To [...] de[...] se[...] wh[...] dis[...] the [...] wh[...] in [...]

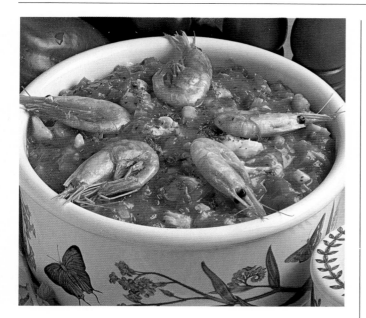

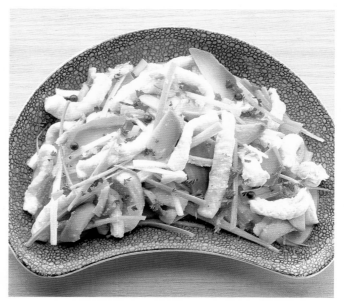

91 | Turbot and Prawn Creole

Preparation time
15 minutes

Cooking time
35-40 minutes

Serves 4

Calories
126 per portion

You will need
1 onion, chopped
1 green pepper, seeded and
    chopped
1 x 400-g/14-oz can tomatoes
½ teaspoon basil
½ teaspoon oregano
pinch of sugar
salt and pepper
250 g/9 oz turbot, cut into cubes
250 g/9 oz peeled, cooked prawns
2 teaspoons cornflour
2 tablespoons dry white wine

For the garnish
whole cooked prawns
chopped parsley

Put the onion, green pepper, tomatoes and their juice, basil, oregano and sugar in a saucepan. Add salt and pepper to taste. Bring to the boil, cover and simmer for 15 minutes.

Add the turbot and prawns and simmer for a further 10-15 minutes. Blend the cornflour and wine until smooth, then stir into the sauce. Heat until the sauce thickens and continue cooking for 2 minutes.

Transfer to a hot serving dish and garnish with whole prawns and chopped parsley.

92 | Stir-fried Crab and Sole

Preparation time
25 minutes

Cooking time
7-10 minutes

Serves 4

Calories
326 per portion

You will need
25 g/1 oz butter
2 tablespoons olive oil
1 small onion, finely chopped
1 garlic clove, crushed
2 leeks, cleaned and cut into
    julienne strips
350 g/12 oz sole fillets, skinned
    and cut into thin strips
225 g/8 oz white crabmeat, flaked
4 tablespoons chicken stock
1 small avocado, peeled, halved,
    stoned and sliced
1 teaspoon grated lemon rind
salt
1 teaspoon green peppercorns in
    brine, drained
2 tablespoons finely chopped
    fresh parsley or dill, to garnish

Heat the butter and oil in a wok or large frying pan and gently fry the onion and garlic for 3 minutes. Add the julienne strips of leek and the strips of sole, and stir-fry gently until the fish is opaque.

Add the crabmeat, stock, avocado slices, lemon rind, salt and peppercorns; stir-fry for 2-3 minutes. Serve immediately, sprinkled with parsley or dill.

Cook's Tip

A less expensive white fish than turbot can be substituted. Supermarkets often reduce the price of peeled, cooked prawns on a Saturday afternoon as they would no longer be fresh on Monday.

Cook's Tip

Wash the leeks thoroughly and dry with absorbent kitchen paper before cutting them into julienne strips. Use a sharp knife to cut even strips about 5 cm/2 inches long.

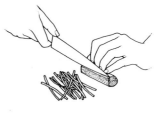

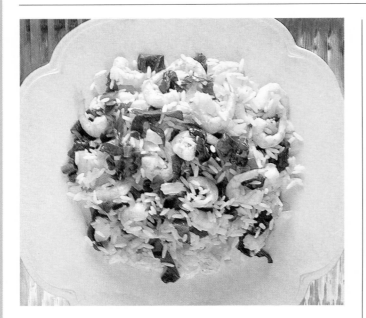

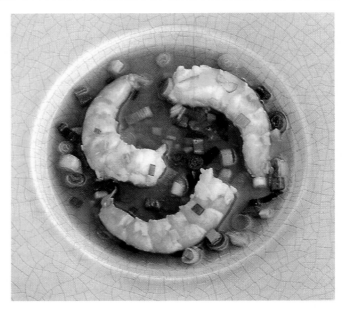

93 | *Prawn and Spinach Pilau*

Preparation time
15 minutes

Cooking time
50-55 minutes

Serves 6

Calories
195 per portion

You will need
750 g/1 lb cooked prawns in their
    shells
2 x 5-cm/2-inch pieces lemon peel
3 parsley sprigs
1 thyme sprig
1 bay leaf
6 white peppercorns, crushed
1.2 litres/2 pints water
750 g/1½ lb spinach
350 g/12 oz long-grain rice
3 tablespoons olive oil
2 large onions, finely chopped
1 garlic clove, crushed
freshly grated nutmeg
Maldon or sea salt

Make the prawn stock (see Cook's Tip). Wash the spinach, then chop off and discard tough stalks. Shred finely. Measure and note the volume of rice, rinse in boiling water and soak in fresh boiled water for 5 minutes.

Heat the oil in a large saucepan, add the onion and cook gently for about 5 minutes, until starting to soften. Add the garlic and spinach, and stir-fry for 2-3 minutes. Drain the rice and add to the pan, stirring until it gleams with a light coating of oil, then grate over a generous amount of nutmeg. Measure out the same volume of prawn stock as the rice and pour over the rice. Season well, bring quickly to the boil, bubble for 10 seconds, then reduce the heat, add the prawns, cover and cook for 15-20 minutes until the liquid is absorbed. Turn off the heat, stir, then cover the pan and leave for 5 minutes.

Cook's Tip

To make the prawn stock, shell the prawns and put their heads and shells into a large pan with the lemon peel, herbs and peppercorns. Add the cold water and bring to the boil, then simmer for 20 minutes. Strain.

94 | *Prawns in Ginger Sauce*

Preparation time
10 minutes

Cooking time
6-7 minutes

Serves 4

Calories
30 per portion

You will need
8 spring onions, chopped
1 x 5-cm/2-inch piece fresh root
    ginger, chopped
2 tablespoons dry sherry
2 tablespoons soy sauce
150 ml/¼ pint chicken stock
salt and pepper
12 peeled, cooked Mediterranean
    prawns

Put all the ingredients, except the prawns, in a saucepan, seasoning with salt and pepper to taste. Bring to the boil, then simmer for 2 minutes.

Stir in the prawns, cover and cook for 3 minutes. Serve immediately.

Cook's Tips

Noodles are the traditional accompaniment to this dish. Cook some fresh egg noodles for 1 minute in boiling salted water. If using the dried variety, cook according to the instructions on the packet.

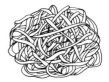

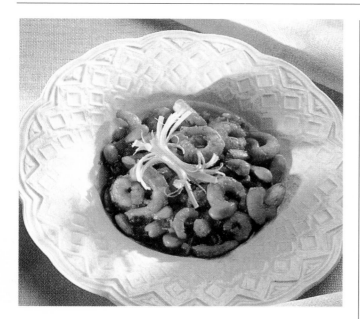

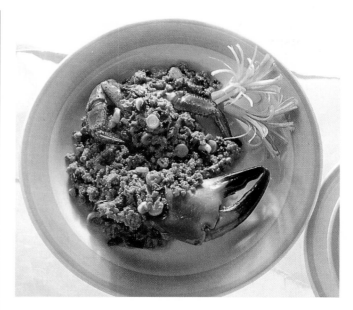

95 | Prawns with Almonds

Preparation time
25 minutes

Cooking time
4-6 minutes

Serves 4

Calories
232 per portion

You will need
75 g/3 oz blanched almonds
350 g/12 oz peeled, cooked
    prawns
2 teaspoons cornflour
1 teaspoon finely chopped fresh
    root ginger
1 small garlic clove, crushed
2 tablespoons oil
1 celery stick, finely chopped
2 teaspoons soy sauce
2 teaspoons dry sherry
2 tablespoons water
pepper
spring onion flowers, to garnish

Brush a frying pan lightly with oil, add the almonds, then heat and toss until golden; be careful not to let them burn. Drain on absorbent kitchen paper.

Put the prawns in a basin with the cornflour, ginger and garlic and mix well. Heat the oil in the frying pan, add the prawn mixture and celery and stir-fry for 2-3 minutes. Add the soy sauce, sherry, water and pepper, and bring to the boil. Add the toasted almonds and heat for 30 seconds, stirring.

Garnish with spring onion flowers (see Recipe 96) and serve hot.

96 | Crab in Black Bean Sauce

Preparation time
35 minutes

Cooking time
12-15 minutes

Serves 4

Calories
345 per portion

You will need
2 tablespoons oil
2 tablespoons salted black beans,
    coarsely chopped
2 garlic cloves, crushed
2 tablespoons finely chopped root
    ginger
4 spring onions, chopped
250 g/9 oz lean pork, finely
    minced
1 large cooked crab, cut into
    pieces
2 tablespoons dry sherry
300 ml/½ pint chicken stock
2 eggs, beaten
1-2 teaspoons sesame oil
spring onion flowers, to garnish
(see Cook's Tip)

Heat the oil in a wok or large frying pan, add the black beans, garlic, ginger and spring onions and stir-fry briskly for 30 seconds. Add the pork and brown quickly for 1 minute. Add the crab, sherry and stock and boil rapidly for 8-10 minutes.

Combine the eggs and sesame oil and stir into the wok. Stir for 30 seconds, until the egg has cooked into strands. Transfer to a warmed serving dish, garnish with spring onion flowers and serve immediately.

Cook's Tip

Serve a stir-fried vegetable such as Stir-fried Chinese Leaves (recipe 189) with this dish. Noodles or plain boiled rice would also make suitable accompaniments.

Cook's Tip

To make spring onion flowers, trim the green top and remove the white part. Shred the top, leaving 2.5 cm/1 inch attached at the base. Immerse in iced water until the spring onion opens out and curls (about 1 hour).

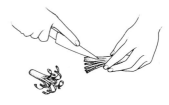

Meat

A cosmopolitan choice of recipes from many different countries is provided in this chapter. Classic French dishes such as Côtes de Porc Vallée d'Auge have been adapted for the calorie-conscious. Many of the recipes show how very successfully fruit and meat can be combined. There are plenty of wholesome casseroles for feeding the family as well as more sophisticated dishes for special occasions. There are recipes using beef, pork, lamb, veal and kidneys as well as liver which, with its high iron content, makes a valuable contribution to a healthy diet.

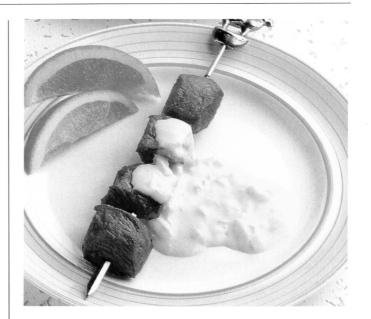

97 | Cutlets with Tarragon

Preparation time
25 minutes

Cooking time
25 minutes

Serves 4

Calories
479 per portion

You will need
50 g/2 oz butter
2 shallots, very finely chopped
250 g/9 oz button mushrooms, very finely chopped
8 lamb cutlets, trimmed
salt and pepper
150 ml/¼ pint dry white wine
2 tablespoons chopped tarragon
½ teaspoon Dijon mustard
8 artichoke hearts, steamed and sprinkled with lemon juice
tarragon sprigs, to garnish

Melt the butter in a saucepan, add the shallots and cook for 5 minutes. Add the mushrooms, cover and cook for 1 minute. Remove the lid and cook rapidly for 2 minutes; set aside.

Season the cutlets with salt and pepper and brown quickly on both sides in a hot frying pan or wok, then cook for 4 minutes on each side. Remove and keep hot. Add the wine to the pan and stir well. Add half the tarragon and the mustard, bring to the boil and cook rapidly for 5 minutes, until reduced by half. Return the cutlets and heat through.

Arrange the cutlets on a warmed serving dish. Spoon the sauce over the meat and sprinkle with the remaining tarragon. Garnish with the artichoke hearts stuffed with the mushroom mixture and tarragon sprigs. Serve immediately.

Cook's Tip

Steaming is the best way to heat the artichoke hearts. Just arrange them on a plate and lower this carefully into the top of the steamer before putting this over a pan of gently bubbling water.

98 | Skewered Lamb

Preparation time
20 minutes, plus marinating

Cooking time
10 minutes

Serves 4

Calories
347 per portion

You will need
450 g/1 lb lamb fillet, cut into 2.5 cm/1 inch cubes
¼ teaspoon crushed black peppercorns
salt
150 ml/¼ pint dry white wine
coarsely grated rind of ½ orange
pinch of ground cinnamon
1 small onion, thinly sliced

For the sauce
1 small onion, finely chopped
1 tablespoon olive oil
pinch of saffron strands
1 egg yolk
2 tablespoons natural low-fat yogurt
juice of ½ orange
1 teaspoon cornflour
artificial liquid sweetener, to taste

Put the cubed lamb into a shallow dish with the peppercorns, salt, white wine, orange rind, cinnamon and sliced onion. Cover and chill for 2 hours. Drain the meat, reserving the marinade and thread on to skewers. Grill the kebabs under a preheated grill 4-5 minutes each side.

Meanwhile make the sauce. Fry the chopped onion in the olive oil for 3 minutes. Add the strained marinade and the saffron and bubble briskly for 1 minute. Blend the egg yolk with the yogurt, orange juice and cornflour; add to the sauce and stir over a gentle heat until lightly thickened. Add a little artificial sweetener if necessary.

Serve the cooked kebabs accompanied by the sauce.

Cook's Tip

Saffron comes from the dried flower pistils of a variety of crocus. As you would need about 60,000 of the pistils to produce 450 g/1 lb of saffron, it is not really practical to try growing it in your herb garden!

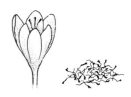

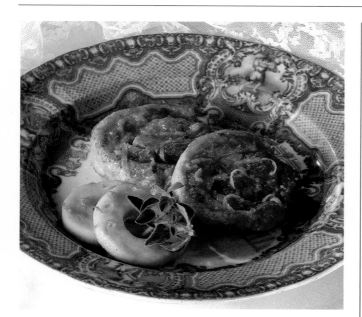

99 | Lamb with Apple Rings

Preparation time
10 minutes, plus
soaking

Cooking time
20-25 minutes

Serves 4

Calories
575 per portion

You will need
8 small noisettes of lamb,
   trimmed of excess fat
2 tablespoons wholemeal flour
freshly ground black pepper
½ teaspoon dried oregano
150 ml/¼ pint chicken stock
1 teaspoon grated orange rind
2 tablespoons orange juice
8 dried apple rings, soaked for 1-2
   hours and drained
salt
sprigs of oregano, to garnish

Dry the lamb and toss it in the flour seasoned with pepper and oregano. Place the noisettes in a non-stick frying pan over a moderate heat and cook for about 3 minutes on each side until they are evenly browned. Reduce the heat and cook them for about 10 minutes, turning them once, until they are cooked the way you like them. Transfer the noisettes to a warmed serving dish and keep them warm. Wipe the frying pan with absorbent kitchen paper to remove any traces of fat.

Add the stock, orange rind, orange juice and apple rings to the pan, season with salt and pepper and bring to the boil. Lower the heat and simmer fo 5 minutes, or until the apple rings are just tender.

Pour the sauce over the lamb, arrange the apple rings and garnish with the oregano.

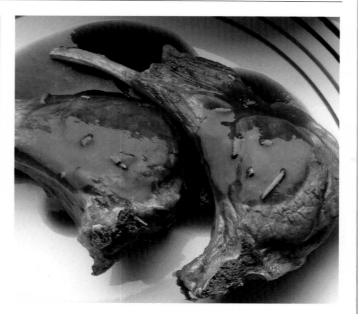

100 | Lamb with Piquant Sauce

Preparation time
15 minutes, plus
marinating

Cooking time
10-15 minutes

Serves 4

Calories
349 per portion

You will need
8 lamb cutlets, trimmed
2 beef stock cubes
8 tablespoons Worcestershire
   sauce
2 teaspoons chopped fresh
   rosemary
1 teaspoon ground coriander
120 ml/4 fl oz water
salt and pepper

Put the cutlets in a flameproof dish. Crumble the stock cubes into the Worcestershire sauce and stir in the rosemary and coriander. Pour over the lamb and leave to marinate for at least 3 hours, turning frequently.

Remove the lamb from the marinade and cook under a hot grill for 10 minutes, or until the lamb is cooked to your taste. Turn the meat frequently, spooning over some of the marinade to prevent burning.

Put the remaining marinade in a saucepan with the water, salt and pepper, and bring to the boil. Arrange the lamb cutlets on a heated serving dish and pour the sauce over.

Cook's Tip

If you happen to have a lot of cooking apples, you can, of course, use these instead of dried apple rings. Just peel, core and cut into slices about 5 mm/¼ inch thick. The cooking time will depend on the type of apple.

Cook's Tip

Stock cubes tend to be very salty, so add the minimum of salt to the marinade. Study the labels to check the contents of the stock cubes and avoid those with additives.

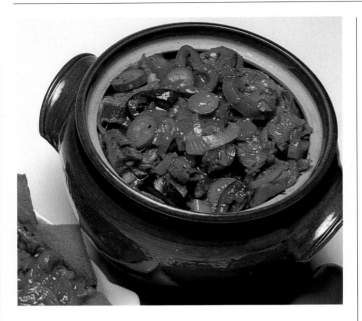

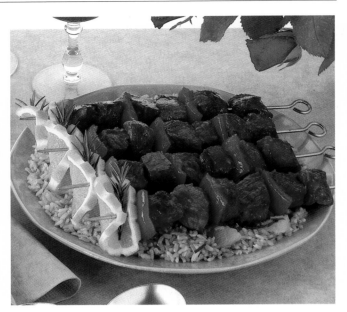

101 | Lamb Ratatouille

Preparation time
25 minutes, plus
draining

Cooking time
1¼ hours

Oven temperature
180°C, 350°F, gas 4

Serves 6

Calories
291 per portion

You will need
1 large aubergine, halved
lengthways and sliced
salt and pepper
1 tablespoon olive oil
1 kg/2¼ lb boned shoulder of
lamb, cubed
1 large onion, sliced
750 g/1½ lb courgettes, sliced
½ green pepper, seeded and
sliced
1-400-g/14-oz can tomatoes
1 teaspoon dried basil

Sprinkle the aubergine slices with salt and leave to drain for 30 minutes. Rinse and pat the slices dry with absorbent kitchen paper.

Put the lamb cubes in a deep non-stick frying pan over a moderate heat and brown on all sides, then remove and set aside.

Add the onion to the pan with the oil and fry until softened. Add the aubergine, courgettes, red and green peppers, tomatoes with their juice, basil and salt and pepper to taste. Cover and cook for 10 minutes.

Stir the lamb cubes into the vegetable mixture. Cover again and cook in the oven for 1 hour, or until tender.

102 | Paprika and Orange Lamb

Preparation time
20 minutes, plus
marinating

Cooking time
15-20 minutes

Oven temperature
190°C, 375°F, gas 5

Serves 4

Calories
316 per portion

You will need
500 g/1¼ lb lamb fillet, cut into 2.5
cm/1 inch cubes
1 large red pepper, seeded and
cut into 2.5 cm/1 inch pieces

For the marinade
1 tablespoon olive oil
2 tablespoons tomato purée
1 teaspoon paprika
2 tablespoons red wine
1 small onion, grated
grated rind and juice of 1 small
orange
2 teaspoons honey
3 drops Tabasco
salt and pepper

For the garnish
4 rosemary sprigs
4 orange slices

Put the lamb cubes in a shallow dish. Combine the marinade ingredients in a bowl. Pour over the lamb and stir. Cover and refrigerate for 6-8 hours or overnight.

Arrange the lamb on four kebab skewers with the pepper pieces. Place on a rack over a dish or tin and spoon the remaining marinade over the kebabs. Place rosemary sprigs below the kebabs and cook in the oven for 20-30 minutes, or under a preheated medium hot grill for 15-20 minutes, turning once. Put on a heated serving dish, garnish with rosemary sprigs and orange slices.

Cook's Tip

You should carefully trim away all the fat from the shoulder of lamb before cutting it into cubes. Lamb contains quite a lot of invisible fat so it is easy to brown in a dry non-stick pan.

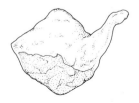

Cook's Tip

Rosemary is an ideal herb to use with lamb. Try adding a couple of sprigs of the herb to the marinade to give the meat a subtle and delicious fragrance. For a more pronounced orange flavour, cut an orange into slices and **alternate with the pieces of pepper on the skewer.**

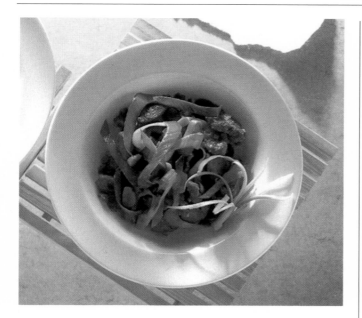

103 | Stir-fried Garlic Lamb

Preparation time
15 minutes, plus marinating

Cooking time
5 minutes

Serves 4

Calories
249 per portion

You will need
350 g/12 oz lamb fillet
2 tablespoons dry sherry
2 tablespoons light soy sauce
1 tablespoon dark soy sauce
1 teaspoon sesame oil
1 tablespoon oil
6 garlic cloves, thinly sliced
1×1-cm/½-inch piece fresh root
    ginger, finely chopped
1 leek, thinly sliced diagonally
4 spring onions, chopped
spring onion flowers, to garnish
    (see Recipe 96)

Cut the lamb into thin slices across the grain. Combine the sherry, soy sauces and sesame oil, add the lamb and toss until well coated. Leave to marinate for 15 minutes, then drain, reserving the marinade.

Heat the oil in a non-stick frying pan, add the meat and about 2 teaspoons of the marinade and fry briskly for about 2 minutes, until well browned. Add the garlic, ginger, leek and spring onions and fry for a further 3 minutes.

Transfer to a warmed serving plate, garnish with the spring onion flowers and serve immediately.

Cook's Tip

This recipe originated in the northern part of China where fresh vegetables are difficult to obtain in the bitterly cold winter months. The lamb is always cooked in a wok there but a frying pan is a satisfactory substitute.

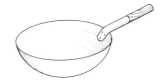

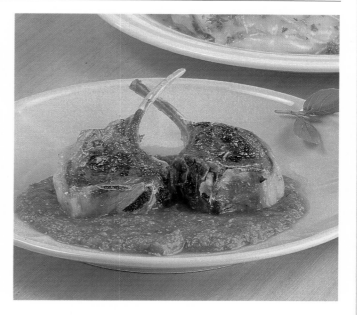

104 | Lamb Cutlets Provençal

Preparation time
20 minutes, plus marinating

Cooking time
15 minutes

Serves 4

Calories
407 per portion

You will need
8 lamb cutlets, trimmed
2 teaspoons olive oil
3 tablespoons red wine
salt and pepper
1 tablespoon chopped fresh basil
1 red pepper, seeded and
    chopped
6 tomatoes, peeled, seeded and
    chopped
4 courgettes, chopped
1 small onion, finely chopped
300 ml/½ pint chicken stock
1 garlic clove, crushed
1 tablespoon tomato purée
fresh basil, to garnish

Put the lamb cutlets into a shallow dish with the olive oil, wine, salt and pepper to taste and the chopped basil; cover and chill for 4 hours.

Put the red pepper, tomatoes, courgettes and onion into a saucepan with the chicken stock, garlic, tomato purée and salt and pepper to taste; simmer gently until the vegetables are just tender.

Drain the marinade from the lamb cutlets; blend the marinade and vegetable sauce in a liquidizer until smooth. Cook the lamb cutlets under a preheated grill for 2-3 minutes on each side. Heat the sauce through.

Spoon a pool of vegetable sauce on to four plates and carefully arrange two cutlets on top of each. Garnish with sprigs of basil and serve.

Cook's Tip

If preferred, the sauce can be served separately, rather than spooned on to each plate. The mixture of tomatoes, courgettes and red pepper with basil is typically Provençal.

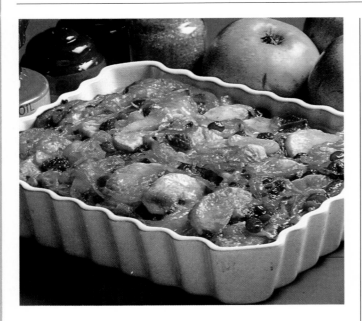

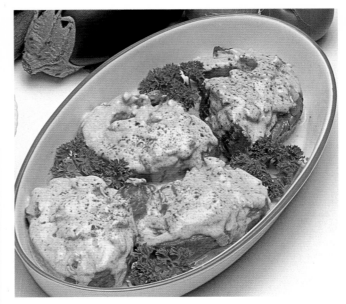

105 | Somerset Lamb Chops

Preparation time
15 minutes

Cooking time
1¾ hours

Oven temperature
180°C, 350°F, gas 4

Serves 4

Calories
466 per portion

You will need
15 g/½ oz butter
1 large onion, thinly sliced
2 large cooking apples, peeled,
   cored and sliced
2 tablespoons raisins
salt and pepper
8 lamb chops, trimmed
150 ml/¼ pint dry cider

Melt the butter in a non-stick frying pan. Add the onion and fry until softened. Remove the onion from the pan with a slotted spoon and spread half over the bottom of a casserole. Cover with half the apple slices and sprinkle with half the raisins, and salt and pepper to taste.

Put the chops in the frying pan and brown on both sides. Drain the chops and place in the casserole. Cover with the remaining onion and apples and sprinkle with the remaining raisins, salt and pepper. Pour in the cider. Cover the casserole and cook in the oven for 1½ hours, or until the chops are very tender.

106 | Paprika Lamb

Preparation time
15 minutes, plus
marinating

Cooking time
1¼ hours

Oven temperature
190°C, 375°F, gas 5

Serves 4

Calories
233 per portion

You will need
4 lamb chops, trimmed
1 onion, finely chopped
150 ml/¼ pint natural low-fat
   yogurt
2 teaspoons paprika

For the marinade
2 tablespoons dry white wine
2 teaspoons lemon juice
½ teaspoon sugar
½ teaspoon dried thyme
salt and pepper

For the garnish
paprika
parsley sprigs

Mix together the marinade ingredients, with salt and pepper to taste. Place the chops in the marinade and leave for 2-3 hours.

Drain the chops and dry with absorbent kitchen paper. Place them in a shallow ovenproof dish. Sprinkle the onion over the chops and cover with foil. Cook in the oven for 1 hour.

Mix the yogurt with the paprika and spoon over the chops. Continue cooking for a further 15 minutes. Serve sprinkled with paprika and garnished with parsley.

Cook's Tip

Pork chops can be cooked in exactly the same way. Both pork and lamb chops should be carefully trimmed to remove as much fat as possible before they are browned. Serve with a crisp green side salad.

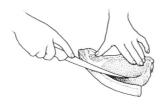

Cook's Tip

This way of cooking lamb chops is based on a typical Hungarian recipe but natural low-fat yogurt is far lower in calories than the traditional soured cream. For a richer sauce, try combining some smetana with the yogurt.

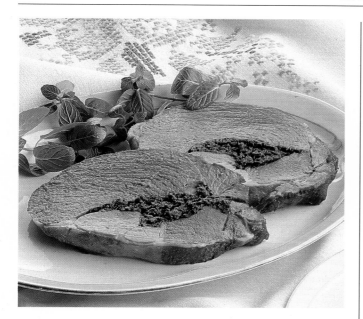

107 | Spinach-stuffed Lamb

Preparation time
20 minutes

Cooking time
45-55 minutes

Oven temperature
180°C, 350°F, gas 4

Serves 4

Calories
154 per portion

You will need
225 g/8 oz fresh or frozen spinach, cooked, drained thoroughly and chopped
15 g/½ oz fresh mint, finely chopped
4 garlic cloves, finely chopped
1 teaspoon vinegar
pinch of sugar
salt and pepper
½ small boned leg of lamb (knuckle end), about 400 g/ 14 oz
175 ml/6 fl oz red wine
fresh mint sprigs, to garnish

Mix the spinach with the mint, garlic, vinegar, sugar and add salt and pepper to taste.

Trim every scrap of fat off the lamb. Lay it out flat with the boned side up and spread the spinach mixture over. Fold the meat over and secure with string as if tying a parcel. Lay the meat in a roasting dish or pan and pour over the red wine, adding a little water if the pan is much larger than the meat. Cook in the oven for 45-55 minutes.

Transfer to a hot carving platter and cut into thick slices. Pour off the excess fat from the roasting pan and pour the remaining juices over the lamb slices. Serve immediately with rice, garnishing the lamb with fresh mint.

Cook's Tip

Ask the butcher to remove the bone but do not let him roll the lamb. The piece of meat should be roughly triangular. The cooking time depends on whether you like lamb well cooked or slightly pink.

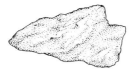

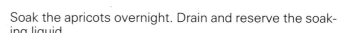

108 | Shoulder of Lamb Stuffed with Apricots

Preparation time
20 minutes, plus soaking

Cooking time
1½ hours

Oven temperature
200°C, 400°F, gas 6

Serves 6

Calories
431 per portion

You will need
175 g/6 oz dried apricots
25 g/1 oz chopped onion
2 teaspoons chopped fresh rosemary or 1 teaspoon dried rosemary
75 g/3 oz wholemeal breadcrumbs
1 egg, beaten
salt and pepper
1 x 1.5 kg/3 lb shoulder of lamb, boned

Soak the apricots overnight. Drain and reserve the soaking liquid.

Roughly chop the apricots, add the onion, rosemary and breadcrumbs. Add the beaten egg to the mixture to bind. Add a little apricot soaking liquid, if necessary, and salt and pepper to taste.

Spoon the stuffing into the lamb bone cavity and sew up the edges, using a trussing needle and string, to enclose the stuffing completely. Roast in the oven for 1½ hours, or until tender.

Cook's Tip

If any meat remains on a joint after the meal, the joint should be put on a clean plate as the juices sour quickly and would spoil the meat. You could save preparation time by using no-soak dried apricots.

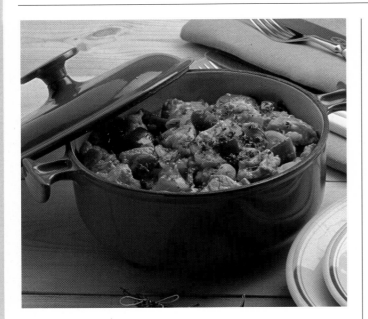

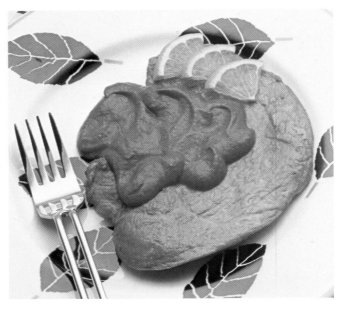

109 | Italian Veal Casserole

Preparation time
20 minutes

Cooking time
1¼-1¾ hours

Oven temperature
180°C, 350°F, gas 4

Serves 2

Calories
301 per portion

You will need
1 tablespoon oil
350 g/12 oz lean veal, cubed
1 garlic clove, crushed
1 small onion, sliced
½ green pepper, seeded and
  chopped
150 g/5 oz tomatoes, peeled and
  chopped
200 ml/7 fl oz light stock
salt and pepper
bouquet garni
chopped parsley, to garnish

Heat the oil in a frying pan, add the veal and fry, turning, until golden brown all over. Add the garlic and onion and cook until they are soft.

Stir in the green pepper, tomatoes, stock and salt and pepper to taste. Transfer to a 1.2 litre/2 pint casserole. Add the bouquet garni. Cover and cook in the oven for 1¼-1½ hours.

Remove the bouquet garni and skim off any excess fat. Serve hot, garnished with parsley.

110 | Veal Paprika

Preparation time
10 minutes

Cooking time
10 minutes

Serves 4

Calories
251 per portion

You will need
4 veal fillets, about 175 g/6 oz
  each
1 tablespoon lemon juice
4 tablespoons tomato purée
3 teaspoons paprika
300 ml/½ pint natural low-fat
  yogurt
salt and pepper

Put the veal fillets on the rack of a grill pan. Cook under a fairly hot grill for about 5 minutes on each side (depending on the thickness of the fillets), spooning over some of the lemon juice to prevent the meat burning.

Mix together the tomato purée, paprika and remaining lemon juice and heat gently. Remove from the heat and stir in the yogurt and salt and pepper to taste.

Put the veal fillets on a warmed serving plate and pour the sauce over.

Cook's Tip

A classic bouquet garni consists of parsley stalks, bay leaves and thyme sprigs. There is much more flavour in the parsley stalks than in the decorative leaves. Tie the herbs securely in a piece of butter muslin.

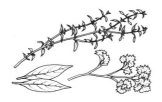

Cook's Tip

This sauce has a rather sharp taste. If you prefer a slightly sweeter sauce, use fresh orange juice instead of the lemon juice. Alternatively, you could add a few drops of artifical liquid sweetener just before serving.

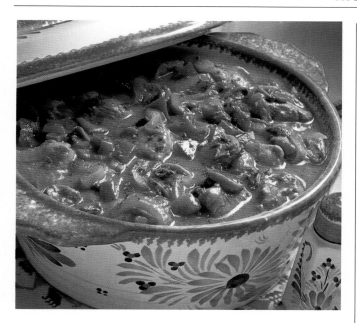

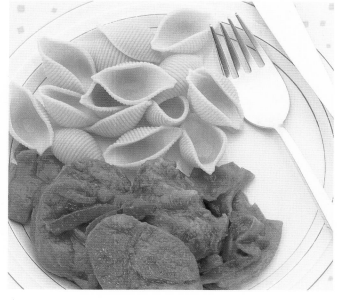

111 | *Hungarian Veal*

Preparation time
20 minutes

Cooking time
1¼-1¾ hours

Oven temperature
180°C, 350°F, gas 4

Serves 4

Calories
226 per portion

You will need
1 tablespoon oil
500 g/1¼ lb lean veal, cut into
  cubes
1 onion, sliced
3 teaspoons paprika
1 green pepper, seeded and
  chopped
50 g/2 oz button mushrooms,
  sliced
300 ml/½ pint tomato juice
85 ml/3 fl oz beef stock
½ teaspoon sugar
salt and pepper
grated nutmeg
1 bay leaf
4 tablespoons natural low-fat
  yogurt
chopped parsley, to garnish

Heat the oil in a large frying pan, add the veal and fry for 5 minutes. Add the onion and fry for 2-3 minutes. Stir in the paprika and cook for 1 minute. Add the green pepper, mushrooms, tomato juice, stock, sugar, salt, pepper and nutmeg to taste, and the bay leaf. Bring to the boil, stirring, then transfer to a 1.75 litre/3 pint casserole.

Cook in the oven for 1-1½ hours. Stir in the yogurt just before serving. Garnish with chopped parsley.

112 | *Veal Pörkölt*

Preparation time
15 minutes

Cooking time
1 hour

Serves 6

Calories
413 per portion

You will need
750 g/1½ lb pie veal in one piece
25 g/1 oz pure lard
2 large onions, finely chopped
1 tablespoon sweet paprika
½ teaspoon salt
1 tablespoon water
1 green pepper, halved and
  seeded
1 large tomato, halved
450 g/1 lb pasta shells or noodles,
  cooked

Cut the meat into large pieces of about 5 cm/2 inches.

Heat the lard in a heavy-based saucepan and fry the onions until golden. Take the pan off the heat and add the paprika, stir thoroughly, then add the meat and return to a gentle heat. Stir and add the salt and the water. Cover and simmer slowly, stirring from time to time and adding a little more water should it look at all dry. After 30 minutes add the halved green pepper and tomato, cover and continue cooking until the meat is really tender; the longer and slower the better.

Just before serving, remove the green pepper, chop up and combine with the veal. Turn the pörkölt into a large warmed serving dish and surround with pasta shells or noodles.

Cook's Tip

For an authentic flavour, use genuine rose paprika. This popular spice is obtainable from some Middle European delicatessens in several different strengths, depending on which portion of the capsicum pod was used.

Cook's Tip

If possible, use a boned knuckle of veal which is the ideal joint for this Hungarian dish. Traditionally, pure lard is used to fry the onions but 1-2 tablespoons of olive oil may be substituted.

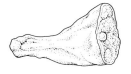

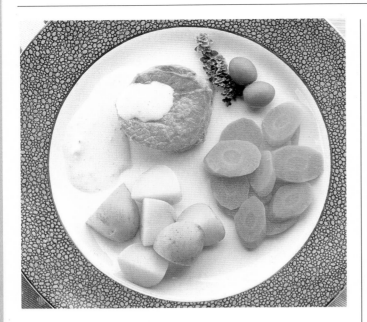

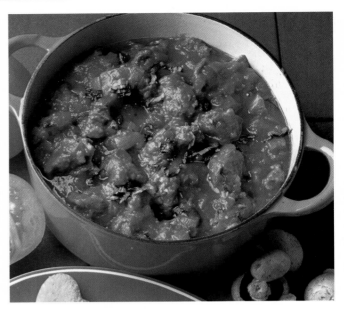

113 | Veal with Olives

Preparation time
15 minutes

Cooking time
30-35 minutes

Serves 4

Calories
305 per portion

You will need
1 tablespoon olive oil
4 veal noisettes, trimmed of fat, about 150 g/5 oz each
1 small onion, thinly sliced
1 bay leaf
1 strip of lemon rind
300 ml/½ pint dry white wine
50 g/2 oz green olives, stoned and finely chopped
1 teaspoon fresh thyme
salt and pepper
3 tablespoons natural low-fat yogurt
1 egg yolk

For the garnish
8 large green olives
sprigs of fresh thyme

Heat the olive oil in a non-stick frying pan and gently fry the noisettes until lightly golden. Add the onion, bay leaf, lemon rind, white wine, stoned green olives and thyme with salt and pepper to taste. Cover and simmer for 25 minutes, until tender. Remove and keep warm.

Discard the bay leaf and blend the cooking liquid with the yogurt and egg yolk. Heat the sauce through very gently without allowing it to come to the boil.

Spoon the hot sauce over the veal and garnish with the olives and sprigs of thyme.

114 | Sauté de Veau Marengo

Preparation time
30 minutes

Cooking time
2¼ hours

Oven temperature
160°C, 325°F, gas 3

Serves 6

Calories
309 per portion

You will need
1 kg/2¼ lb lean stewing veal
wholemeal flour for coating
salt and pepper
1 tablespoon oil
2 onions, chopped
6 tablespoons dry white vermouth
300 ml/½ pint dry white wine
500 g/1 ¼ lb tomatoes, peeled, seeded and chopped
2 tablespoons tomato purée
1 teaspoon chopped basil
1 teaspoon chopped oregano
strip of orange rind
2 garlic cloves, crushed
250 g/9 oz button mushrooms
chopped basil, to garnish (optional)

Cut the veal into 2.5 cm/1 inch cubes. Season the flour with salt and pepper and use to coat the veal lightly.

Heat the oil in a non-stick frying pan, add the veal and fry until browned on all sides. Transfer to a flameproof casserole. Add the onion to the pan and fry until golden. Add to the casserole, with the remaining ingredients. Bring to the boil, then cook in the oven for about 2 hours, until tender. Remove the orange rind.

Garnish with basil, if using.

Cook's Tip

Pare the lemon carefully to ensure no pith is attached to the rind. In some Greek delicatessens it is possible to buy fresh olives. If you use ones that have been preserved in brine, rinse thoroughly in cold water.

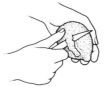

Cook's Tip

For a more economical version of this dish, replace the white wine with chicken or veal stock. The dry white vermouth gives a distinctive flavour. Serve with some plain boiled noodles.

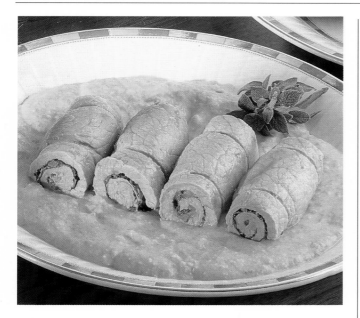

115 | Veal Paupiettes

Preparation time
20 minutes

Cooking time
20-25 minutes

Serves 4

Calories
293 per portion

You will need
4 veal escalopes, flattened, about
   150 g/5 oz each
1 teaspoon grated lemon rind
1 small onion, chopped
freshly ground black pepper
1 tablespoon chopped sage
4 large lettuce leaves
20 g/¾ oz butter
1 tablespoon olive oil
150 ml/¼ pint dry white wine
150 ml/¼ pint chicken stock
2 parsnips, peeled, chopped and
   cooked
2 tablespoons natural low-fat
   yogurt
2 canned red pimentos
1 tablespoon chopped chives
salt

Sprinkle the escalopes with the lemon rind, onion, pepper and sage. Lay a lettuce leaf on top of each and roll up. Tie neatly with fine string.

Heat the butter and oil in a shallow pan; add the prepared veal paupiettes and cook until evenly coloured on all sides. Add the wine and chicken stock; cover and simmer until the veal is tender.

Meanwhile, blend the parsnips, yogurt and red pimentos in a liquidizer. Mix in the chives and season. Heat through in a double saucepan.

Spoon the purée on to a warmed serving dish and arrange the paupiettes on top.

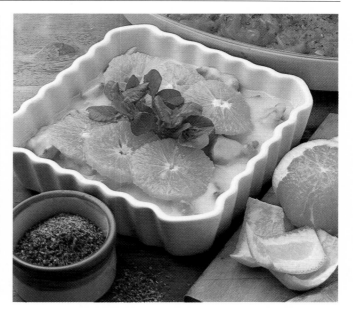

116 | Veal with Orange

Preparation time
25 minutes

Cooking time
1¾-2¼ hours

Oven temperature
180°C, 350°F, gas 4

Serves 4

Calories
304 per portion

You will need
1 tablespoon oil
750 g/1½ lb lean pie veal, cubed
1 onion, sliced
3 tablespoons wholemeal flour
300 ml/½ pint chicken stock
150 ml/¼ pint unsweetened
   orange juice
salt and pepper
2 oranges, peeled and sliced
watercress, to garnish

Heat the oil in a non-stick frying pan. Add the veal cubes and brown on all sides. Transfer with a slotted spoon to a casserole. Add the onion to the pan and fry until golden brown. Add to the casserole.

Stir the flour into the fat remaining in the pan and cook for 3 minutes. Gradually stir in the stock and orange juice and bring to the boil. Season with salt and pepper to taste. Pour over the veal cubes. Arrange the orange slices, overlapping, on top.

Cook in the oven for 1½-2 hours, or until the veal is tender. Garnish with watercress.

Cook's Tip

Use a heavy metal cleaver to flatten the veal escalopes. If you do not have one, an old-fashioned flat iron is a good substitute! If you dip the cleaver in cold water first, this will help to prevent your tearing the veal.

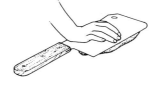

Cook's Tip

Depending on the time of year different varieties of oranges are available. The best types to use in casseroles are those with thin skins, juicy flesh and few pips, such as the Navel and Valencia.

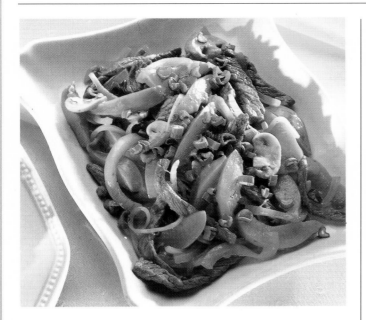

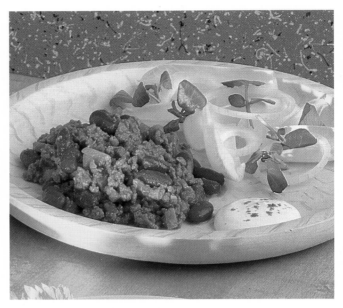

117 | Beef with Plums

Preparation time
20 minutes

Cooking time
10 minutes

Serves 2

Calories
315 per portion

You will need
1 tablespoon oil
1 onion, thinly sliced
1 garlic clove, crushed
2-3 pieces beef for beef olives,
    cut into thin slivers
2-3 dessert plums, stoned and cut
    into slices
2-3 mushrooms, thinly sliced
1 tablespoon sherry
1 tablespoon soy sauce
2 teaspoons cornflour, blended
    with 2 tablespoons water
chopped spring onion tops, to
    garnish

Heat the oil in a large frying pan, add the onion and fry for 2 minutes. Stir in the garlic, then push the mixture to one side of the pan. Tilt the pan to let the juices run out of the onion and over the base. Scatter in the meat strips and stir-fry over a high heat for 2 minutes, until the meat is evenly coloured.

Lower the heat and add the plums and mushrooms. Continue to stir-fry for 1 minute, then stir in the sherry, soy sauce and blended cornflour. Cook, stirring, until the sauce has thickened.

Garnish with spring onions and serve with wholemeal tagliatelle and green vegetables.

118 | Chilli Beef

Preparation time
20 minutes

Cooking time
30-35 minutes

Serves 4

Calories
380 per portion

You will need
1 tablespoon olive oil
1 small onion, finely chopped
1 garlic clove, crushed
450 g/1 lb lean minced beef
1 tablespoon chilli powder
1 tablespoon tomato purée
300 ml/½ pint beef stock
6 tomatoes, peeled, seeded and
    chopped
1 small red pepper, seeded and
    chopped
1 x 225-g/8-oz can kidney beans,
    rinsed and drained

For the garnish
4 tablespoons natural low-fat
    yogurt
chilli powder (optional)

Heat the oil and fry the onion gently for 3 minutes; add the garlic and beef and fry until browned. Stir in the chilli powder and cook for 1 minute. Add the tomato purée, beef stock, tomatoes, chopped red pepper and kidney beans. Cover and simmer gently for 20-25 minutes, until the minced beef is tender.

Spoon the minced beef on to warmed plates and place a tablespoon of yogurt next to it. Sprinkle a little chilli powder over the yogurt, if liked. Serve immediately with rice or a salad.

Cook's Tip

The beef used for beef olives is sold rolled up in thin raw slices. These are now available in many large supermarkets. Imported plums are often on sale outside our own short season.

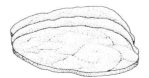

Cook's Tip

If you have not used chilli powder before, it is best to add only 1 teaspoon at first as you may find that 1 tablespoon makes the beef too fiery. It is very much a matter of personal taste.

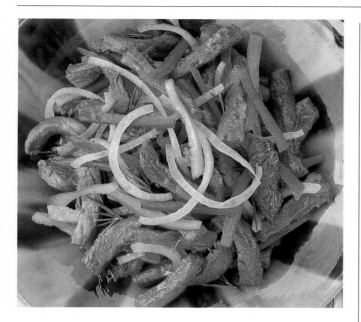

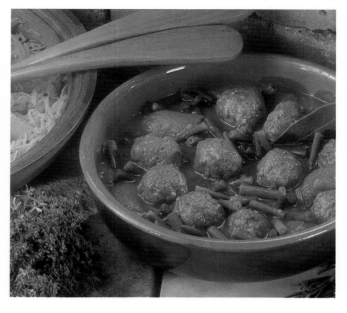

119 | Stir-fried Beef with Peppers

Preparation time
15 minutes

Cooking time
10-12 minutes

Serves 4

Calories
218 per portion

You will need
1 tablespoon olive oil
1 onion, and thinly sliced
1 large garlic clove, cut into thin strips
450 g/1 lb fillet steak, cut into thin strips
1 red pepper, seeded and cut into matchstick strips
1 green pepper, seeded and cut into matchstick strips
1 tablespoon soy sauce
2 tablespoons dry sherry
salt and pepper
1 tablespoon chopped fresh rosemary

Heat the olive oil in a deep frying pan or wok and stir-fry the onion and garlic for 2 minutes. Add the strips of beef and stir-fry briskly until evenly browned on all sides and almost tender. Add the strips of red and green pepper and stir-fry for a further 2 minutes. Add the soy sauce, sherry, salt and pepper to taste and the rosemary, and stir-fry for a further 1-2 minutes.

Serve piping hot with brown rice.

Cook's Tip

Fillet steak is the most suitable cut to use for this dish. Less expensive cuts tend to be tougher and are better suited to slower methods of cooking. You can sometimes buy fillet steak at a reduced price late on a Saturday.

120 | Summer Vegetable Hotpot

Preparation time
20 minutes

Cooking time
35 minutes

Oven temperature
200°C, 400°F, gas 6

Serves 4

Calories
418 per portion

You will need
450 g/1 lb lean minced beef
1 teaspoon coriander seeds
½ teaspoon very coarsely ground black pepper
½ teaspoon cumin seeds
½ teaspoon salt
1 tablespoon red wine vinegar
2 teaspoons oil
3 x 400-g/14-oz cans tomatoes
1 bay leaf
1 dried chilli
1 kg/2¼ lb French beans, chopped into 2 cm/¾ inch lengths
1 tablespoon red wine

Put the minced beef in a bowl and add the coriander, black pepper, cumin seeds, salt and vinegar. Oil your hands lightly and knead the mixture for a minute before forming walnut-sized balls.

Heat the oil in a frying pan and seal the meatballs. Put in a casserole and add the tomatoes, bay leaf and chilli.

Cook in the oven for about 5 minutes, then add the French beans and red wine. Cook, uncovered, for 15-25 minutes, until the beans are just tender.

Cook's Tip

This hotpot can be cooked on a barbecue, provided you have a flameproof casserole that you do not mind blackening a little. Carefully embed the casserole in the hot coal and allow to heat up before adding the oil.

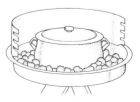

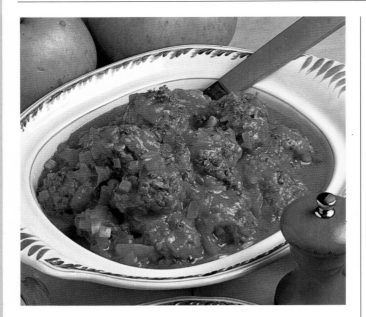

121 | *Meatballs in Tomato Sauce*

Preparation time
15 minutes

Cooking time
45-50 minutes

Serves 4

Calories
349 per portion

You will need
500 g/1¼ lb lean minced beef
1 garlic clove, crushed
1 tablespoon chopped parsley
½ teaspoon cumin seeds
  (optional)
salt and pepper
1 egg, beaten
chopped parsley, to garnish

For the sauce
2 onions, finely chopped
1 x 400-g/14-oz can tomatoes
1 tablespoon tomato purée
½ teaspoon sugar
grated nutmeg

Put the beef, garlic, parsley, cumin seeds (if using) and salt and pepper to taste in a bowl; mix well. Bind the mixture with the egg, then divide into 20 and shape into balls on a floured surface.

Place the sauce ingredients, with nutmeg, salt and pepper to taste, in a large flameproof casserole. Bring to the boil, then lower the heat. Carefully place the meatballs in the liquid, cover and simmer gently for 40-45 minutes, stirring occasionally.

Transfer the meatballs to a warmed serving dish and pour the sauce over. Serve garnished with chopped parsley.

Cook's Tip

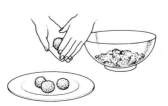

If you dip your fingers in cold water when shaping meatballs, this will help to prevent them becoming sticky and the meat mixture crumbling. Most supermarkets now sell special packs of lean minced beef.

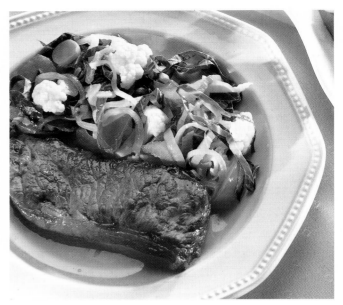

122 | *Steak with Vegetables*

Preparation time
20 minutes

Cooking time
13-15 minutes

Serves 4

Calories
282 per portion

You will need
4 grilling steaks, about 175 g/6 oz
  each
1 tablespoon oil
1 onion, thinly sliced
1 carrot, thinly sliced
2 potatoes, thinly sliced
2 celery sticks, sliced
4-6 spring cabbage or spinach
  leaves, shredded
50 g/2 oz small broccoli or
  cauliflower florets
50 g/2 oz mushrooms, sliced
¼ cucumber, sliced
2-3 tomatoes, cut into wedges
2 tablespoons soy sauce

Cook the steak under a preheated hot grill for 3-5 minutes on each side, depending on thickness and personal taste.

Heat the oil in a large non-stick frying pan, add the onion and fry for 2 minutes. Add the carrot, potato and about 4 tablespoons hot water and stir-fry over a high heat for 3 minutes, using two large wooden spoons to turn the vegetables. Add the celery, cabbage or spinach, and broccoli or cauliflower, and stir-fry for 2 minutes, adding a little more water if necessary to prevent sticking. Add the mushrooms, cucumber and tomatoes and stir-fry for another minute. Add the soy sauce and stir well. The vegetables should be tender but still crisp, with a rich gravy in the bottom of the pan. Serve hot with the steak on warmed plates.

Cook's Tip

Stir-fried vegetables are quick, easy and healthy eating. Always start with an onion, then add any root vegetables and green leaves. Add the softest vegetable last. The vegetable juices will combine to make a nutritious sauce.

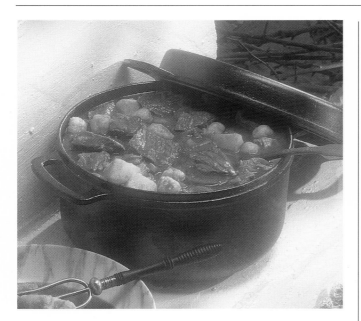

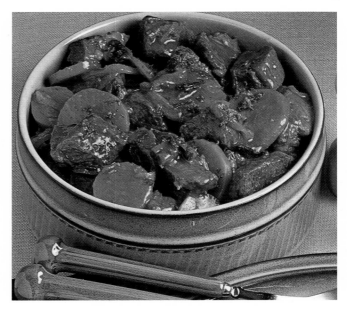

123 | Gulyas

Preparation time
35 minutes

Cooking time
1 hour

Serves 8

Calories
427 per portion

You will need
25 g/1 oz lard
2 large onions, finely chopped
5 teaspoons sweet paprika
1.25 kg/2¾ lb flank steak, cut into 2.5 cm/1 inch cubes
750 g/1½ lb potatoes
1 teaspoon caraway seeds
2 tablespoons tomato purée
2.25 litres/4 pints chicken stock
3 green peppers, seeded, sliced
salt and pepper
175 g/6 oz plain flour
1 egg, lightly beaten

Heat the lard and fry the onions until well coloured. Remove from the heat and add the paprika. Stir well and add the beef, one of the potatoes peeled and grated, and the caraway seeds. Stir and return to the heat, cover and simmer for 10-15 minutes, stirring from time to time.

Add the tomato purée and a cupful of the stock. Cover and simmer until the meat is nearly done. Add the remaining stock. Peel and cube the remaining potatoes and add them with the green peppers as soon as the soup has come to the boil. Cook until the potatoes are done and the meat is tender. Add salt and pepper to taste.

Meanwhile, make the dumplings. Sieve the flour on to a board, make a well in the centre and add the egg and the salt. Work the mixture with your hands into a stiff dough. If this proves impossible, add a drop or two of water. Flatten the dough between the palms of your hands. Pinch off pieces the size of kidney beans and add them to the gulyas 10 minutes before serving.

Cook's Tip

If you have a cast-iron cauldron, you can cook this gulyas (pronounced ghoulash) over a bonfire like the Hungarian vagabonds once did. It is probably much simpler to make on a hob in the kitchen.

124 | Flemish Beef

Preparation time
20 minutes

Cooking time
1¾-2 hours

Oven temperature
180°C, 350°F, gas 4

Serves 4

Calories
296 per portion

You will need
500 g/1¼ lb lean chuck steak, cubed
1 onion, sliced
1 carrot, sliced
1 garlic clove, crushed
75 g/3 oz mushrooms, sliced
300 ml/½ pint light ale
1 beef stock cube
1 teaspoon vinegar
1 teaspoon brown sugar
grated nutmeg
salt and pepper
1 bay leaf
2 teaspoons cornflour
3 tablespoons water
chopped parsley, to garnish

Brown the steak in a non-stick frying pan and place in a 1.75 litre/3 pint casserole. Add the onion, carrot, garlic and mushrooms.

Blend the light ale with the stock cube, vinegar, brown sugar, and nutmeg, salt and pepper to taste. Pour over the meat and vegetables. Add the bay leaf. Cover and cook in the oven for 1½ hours, or until the meat is tender.

Mix the cornflour with the water and stir into the casserole. Cook for 15-20 minutes. Serve garnished with chopped parsley.

Cook's Tip

When you are making a dish such as a casserole that needs a long cooking time, economize on fuel by using the oven to cook another dish at the same time.

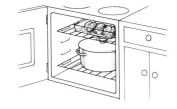

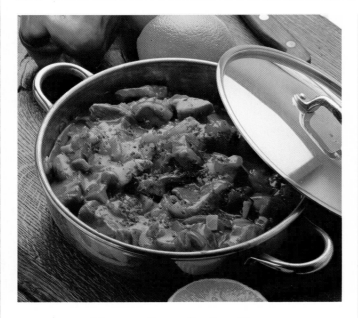

125 | Beef with Orange

Preparation time
20 minutes

Cooking time
1¼-1½ hours

Oven temperature
160°C, 325°F, gas 3

Serves 4

Calories
212 per portion

You will need
5 teaspoons plain wholemeal flour
salt and pepper
350 g/12 oz lean chuck steak,
   cubed
15 g/½ oz butter
1 small onion, chopped
½ green pepper, seeded and
   chopped
grated rind and juice of 2 small
   oranges
200 ml/7 fl oz beef stock
chopped parsley, to garnish

Season the flour with salt and pepper and use to coat the meat. Melt the butter in a non-stick frying pan, add the onion and pepper and fry until soft. Add the meat and fry, turning, until evenly browned. Transfer to a 900 ml/1½ pint casserole.

Stir in the orange rind and juice, stock and salt and pepper to taste. Cover and cook in the oven for 1-1¼ hours. Serve hot, garnished with parsley.

126 | Beef and Artichokes

Preparation time
25 minutes, plus
marinating

Cooking time
1¼ hours

Serves 6

Calories
259 per portion

You will need
1 kg/2¼ lb lean chuck steak, cut
   into cubes
½ teaspoon allspice
½ teaspoon ground cinnamon
½ teaspoon salt
coarsely ground black pepper
4 garlic cloves
8 tablespoons red wine
1 tablespoon oil
½ teaspoon ground cumin
750 g/1½ lb Jerusalem artichokes,
   blanched and scraped, cut into
   chunks

Put the meat in a bowl and sprinkle over the allspice, cinnamon, salt and pepper. Add 2 of the garlic cloves, chopped. Pour over the wine and mix well. Cover and leave to marinate for at least 4 hours (not more than 24).

Heat the oil and fry the remaining garlic, halved, with the cumin. Strain the meat and add to the pan, reserving the marinade. Seal the meat over a high heat, then transfer to a flameproof casserole. Add the artichokes and marinade, cover and simmer for 1 hour.

Cook's Tip

Nothing really compares with the flavour of home-made stock – simmered slowly until it is well reduced and sets in a thick jelly. The fat will have risen to the top and can easily be removed.

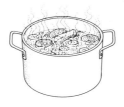

Cook's Tip

The gnarled shapes of Jerusalem artichokes make them rather fiddly to prepare. A potato peeler can be used on the larger artichokes but it is not essential to take the skin off the smaller ones, provided you have scrubbed them thoroughly to remove any traces of earth.

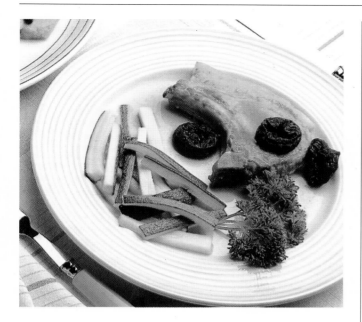

127 | Pork and Prunes

Preparation time
10 minutes, plus
soaking

Cooking time
1¼ hours

Oven temperature
220°C, 425°F, gas 7;
then
160°C, 325°F, gas 3

Serves 4

Calories
192 per portion

You will need
20 prunes, soaked overnight in
  water
4 pork chops, about 175 g/6 oz
  each, trimmed
1 chicken stock cube, crumbled
salt and pepper
1 teaspoon mustard powder
1 tablespoon wine vinegar
parsley sprigs, to garnish

Arrange the prunes in an ovenproof dish. Lay the pork chops on top of the prunes. Add all the remaining ingredients and enough of the prune soaking liquid to cover.

Cook in the oven for 15 minutes, then reduce the temperature and cook for about 1 hour more, or until the chops are tender. Garnish with parsley and serve.

Cook's Tip

Serve this quick-to-prepare casserole with steamed sliced courgettes and plain boiled rice. Rinse the prunes in cold water before leaving them to soak overnight to remove any fragments of leaf.

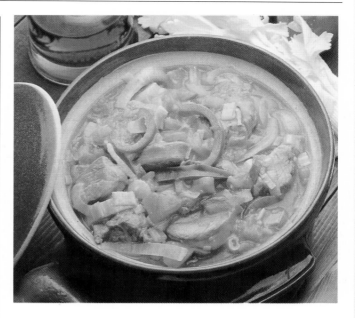

128 | Country Pork Casserole

Preparation time
20 minutes

Cooking time
1¼ hours

Oven temperature
180°C, 350°F, gas 4

Serves 4

Calories
262 per portion

You will need
450 g/1 lb pork fillet
25 g/1 oz flour
salt and pepper
2 tablespoons oil
2 onions, sliced
1-2 leeks, sliced
1-3 celery sticks, diced
1 small green pepper, seeded and
  diced
225 g/8 oz tomatoes, roughly
  chopped
1 tablespoon lemon juice or white
  wine vinegar
150 ml/¼ pint chicken stock
1-2 tablespoons tomato purée

Cut the pork into neat slices. Blend the flour, salt and pepper and use to coat the meat lightly. Heat the oil in a large non-stick frying pan, fry the pork slices on either side until golden brown and transfer to a casserole. Add the onions, leeks and celery to the pan and fry gently for 10 minutes; do not allow the vegetables to brown. Spoon these vegetables over the pork then add the pepper and tomatoes.

Pour the lemon juice or vinegar, chicken stock and tomato purée into the pan; stir well to absorb any meat juices, season to taste, then spoon over the pork and vegetables. Cover the casserole and cook in the oven for 40-50 minutes, or until the meat is tender.

Cook's Tip

The fillet is the leanest cut of pork and also the most tender – it is sometimes called tenderloin. For this dish it is not necessary to buy the fillet in one piece.

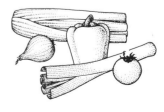

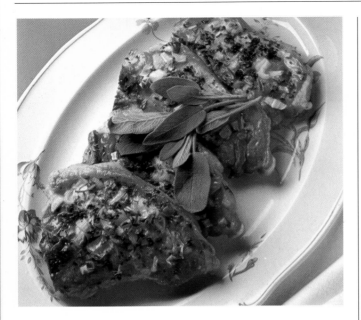

129 | Côtes de Porc Vallée d'Auge

Preparation time
10 minutes

Cooking time
30 minutes

Serves 4

Calories
207 per portion

You will need
4 shallots, chopped
2 tablespoons chopped parsley
salt and pepper
4 pork chops, trimmed
15 g/½ oz butter, melted
150 ml/¼ pint dry cider
sage leaves, to garnish

Mix the shallots and parsley together, with salt and pepper to taste. Score the chops on both sides and spread with the mixture. Spoon over a little melted butter. Cook under a preheated medium grill for about 15 minutes on each side until tender.

Transfer the chops to a frying pan. Drain off any excess fat from the grill pan and pour the juices over the chops. Add the cider and boil for 2 minutes until the liquor has reduced.

Transfer to a warmed serving dish and garnish the chops with sage.

Cook's Tip

For the authentic flavour of this classic French dish, you should use shallots rather than onions. In Normandy a tablespoon of Calvados, the local liqueur, is added just before serving to cut the richness of the pork.

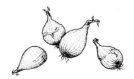

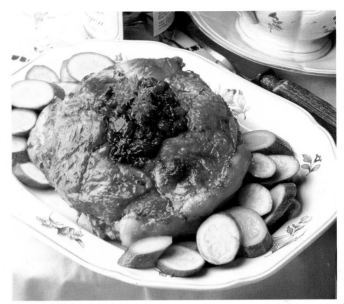

130 | Porc Farci aux Pruneaux

Preparation time
15 minutes, plus soaking

Cooking time
1¾ hours

Oven temperature
190°C, 375°F, gas 5

Serves 6

Calories
388 per portion

You will need
1.5 kg/3 lb piece pork fillet
salt and pepper
175 g/6 oz large prunes
25 g/1 oz seedless raisins
½ teaspoon ground mixed spice
1 tablespoon chopped sage
300 ml/½ pint dry white wine
1 tablespoon redcurrant jelly
150 ml/¼ pint natural low-fat yogurt
parsley sprigs, to garnish

Season the pork with salt and pepper and lay flat. Soak the prunes and raisins in boiling water for 30 minutes. Drain well and stone the prunes.

Mix the spice and sage with the prunes and raisins. Spread over the meat, leaving a 2.5 cm/1 inch border. Roll up and secure with string. Place in a roasting pan and pour over half the wine. Cook in the oven for 1½ hours, or until tender.

Transfer to a warmed serving dish. Add the remaining wine to the roasting pan, place over a low heat and bring to the boil. Simmer for 3-4 minutes until reduced to 150 ml/¼ pint. Add the redcurrant jelly and yogurt, check the seasoning and simmer until thickened.

Garnish the meat with parsley. Serve with steamed courgettes and the sauce.

Cook's Tip

Natural low-fat yogurt has been substituted for the double cream used in the traditional version of this French recipe. The sauce still tastes delicious and is, of course, far less fattening.

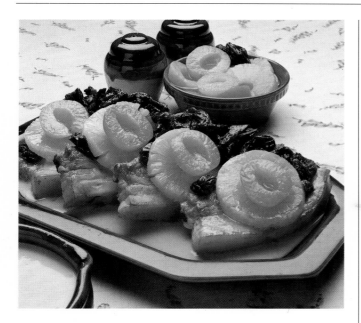

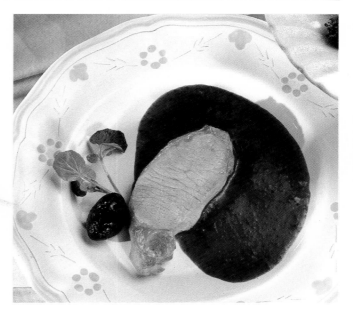

131 | Pork Casserole with Fruit

Preparation time
10 minutes

Cooking time
1¼ hours

Oven temperature
180°C, 350°F, gas 4

Serves 4

Calories
284 per portion

You will need
4 pork chops
1 x 400-g/14-oz can apricot halves
  in natural juice
1 x 225-g/8-oz can pineapple rings
  in natural juice
8 prunes, stoned and chopped
5 tablespoons chicken stock
150 ml/¼ pint natural low-fat
  yogurt
salt and pepper

Put the chops in a frying pan and brown on both sides. Remove the chops from the pan, drain, then arrange in a flameproof casserole.

Drain the apricot halves and pineapple rings, reserving the juice. Place the fruit, with the prunes, on top of the chops to cover them. Mix the stock with 5 tablespoons each of the apricot and pineapple juices. Pour into the casserole. Cover tightly and cook in the oven for about 1 hour or until the chops are tender.

Transfer the chops to a warmed serving dish, being careful not to dislodge the fruit on top. Keep hot.

Boil the liquid in the casserole until reduced to about 150 ml/¼ pint. Skim off any fat, then stir in the yogurt with salt and pepper to taste. Heat through gently and serve this sauce with the pork.

Cook's Tip

If you have time, leave the reduced liquid until cold before skimming off the fat as it is much easier to do then. Alternatively, try using absorbent kitchen paper to mop up the fat.

132 | Pork with Prune Sauce

Preparation time
15 minutes

Cooking time
20 minutes

Serves 4

Calories
316 per portion

You will need
4 pork loin chops, trimmed
1 tablespoon oil
1 small onion, thinly sliced
1 garlic clove, crushed
1 x 400-g/14-oz can prunes in
  natural juice
2 teaspoons cornflour
1 tablespoon soy sauce
2 teaspoons wine vinegar
watercress sprigs, to garnish

Cook the pork under a preheated moderate grill for about 10 minutes on each side, or until cooked through.

Meanwhile, heat the oil in a non-stick frying pan, add the onion and fry for 2 minutes, stirring. Stir in the garlic and set aside.

Drain the prunes, reserving the juice. Remove the stones and set aside 4 prunes for garnish. Put the remaining prunes and the juice in a blender or food processor. Add the cornflour, soy sauce, vinegar and onion mixture and work until smooth. Pour into the pan and cook, stirring, until thick and shiny.

Divide the sauce between warmed individual serving plates and partly lay the grilled pork in it. Garnish with a prune and a watercress sprig.

Cook's Tip

Pork and prunes are a wonderful combination. In this recipe canned prunes in natural juice are used but you can replace these with prunes which have been cooked with water until just tender.

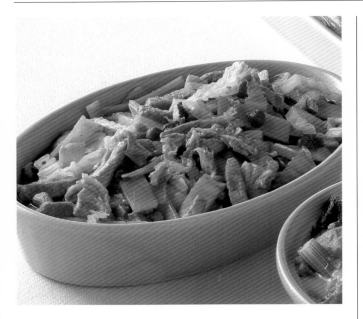

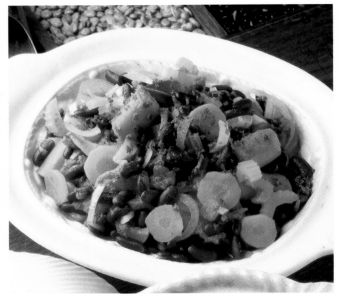

133 | *Chinese Pork with Bamboo Shoots*

Preparation time
15 minutes

Cooking time
20-25 minutes

Serves 4

Calories
203 per portion

You will need
2 tablespoons groundnut oil
300 g/11 oz lean pork, shredded
salt and pepper
1 small Chinese cabbage,
    shredded
1 tablespoon coarsely chopped
    hazelnuts
1×225-g/8-oz can bamboo shoots,
    drained with juices reserved,
    and sliced
2 tablespoons soy sauce
1 teaspoon curry powder
pinch of chilli powder
small pinch of sugar

Heat the oil in a non-stick frying pan or wok, add the pork and stir-fry quickly until lightly browned. Season with salt and pepper to taste. Add the cabbage, hazelnuts and a few tablespoons of the liquid from the can of bamboo shoots. Cook, stirring, for about 5 minutes.

Add the bamboo shoots, soy sauce, curry powder, chilli powder and sugar, mixing well. Cook gently for a further 10 minutes. Serve immediately.

134 | *Black Bean Casserole*

Preparation time
20 minutes, plus
soaking

Cooking time
2½-3 hours

Oven temperature
180°C, 350°F, gas 4

Serves 4

Calories
342 per portion

You will need
400 g/14 oz black beans, soaked
    overnight
1 tablespoon olive oil
2 onions, sliced
2 celery sticks, sliced
2 carrots, sliced
2 garlic cloves, crushed
175 g/6 oz frankfurter sausages,
    sliced
1 tablespoon tomato purée
1 bay leaf
500 g/1¼ lb tomatoes, peeled and
    chopped
salt and pepper
chopped parsley, to garnish

Drain the beans, put in a pan and cover with cold water. Bring to the boil, boil for 10 minutes, then simmer gently for 1 hour. Drain and reserve 450 ml/¾ pint of the liquid.

Heat the oil in a flameproof casserole, add the onions and fry for 5-10 minutes until transparent. Add the celery, carrots and garlic and fry for 3-4 minutes.

Add the remaining ingredients, with the beans, reserved liquid, and salt and pepper to taste. Cover and cook in the oven for 1-1½ hours until the beans are soft. Sprinkle with the parsley and serve immediately.

Cook's Tip

Bamboo shoots are a popular ingredient of many Chinese vegetable dishes. In their native country raw shoots are used but the canned variety is much easier to obtain elsewhere.

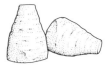

Cook's Tip

It is essential that the black beans are soaked overnight and then cooked exactly as described in the recipe. Try cooking a larger quantity and using the surplus in a salad.

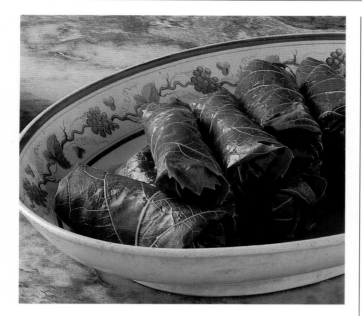

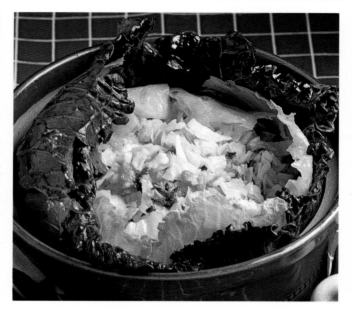

135 | Greek Vine Leaves with Savoury Stuffing

Preparation time
15 minutes

Cooking time
30 minutes

Serves 4

Calories
222 per portion

You will need
1 x 425-g/15-oz can vine leaves
2 tablespoons olive oil
150 g/5 oz lean minced beef
1 large onion, finely chopped
¼ fennel bulb, grated
2 garlic cloves, crushed
150 g/5 oz cooked long-grain rice
1 tablespoon chopped dill
1 teaspoon dried oregano
salt and pepper
150 ml/¼ pint dry red wine
150 ml/¼ pint water
4 tablespoons lemon juice

Put the vine leaves in a sieve, rinse and drain thoroughly.

Heat 1 tablespoon of the oil in a large non-stick frying pan. Add the minced meat, onion, fennel and garlic and fry, stirring, until cooked for about 8-10 minutes. Stir in the rice, dill, oregano and salt and pepper to taste. Spread the mixture evenly over the vine leaves. Fold the long sides of the vine leaves over and roll up securely from the shorter edge to make meat parcels.

Mix the remaining oil, the red wine and water in a saucepan, add the stuffed vine leaves, cover and cook over a gentle heat for about 20 minutes. Remove with a slotted spoon to serve.

136 | Stuffed Cabbage

Preparation time
20 minutes

Cooking time
2 hours

Oven temperature
190°C, 375°F, gas 5

Serves 8

Calories
70 per portion

You will need
1 medium cabbage
1 tablespoon olive oil
4 back bacon rashers, derinded and chopped
1 onion, chopped
1 garlic clove, crushed
1 egg, beaten
2 tablespoons grated Parmesan cheese
3 tablespoons chopped parsley
salt and pepper
250 ml/8 fl oz chicken stock

Cook the whole cabbage in boiling water for 15 minutes. Drain and cool under cold running water. Cut out the core, then remove the inner cabbage leaves, leaving the outside leaves intact. Chop the inner leaves.

Heat the oil in a non-stick frying pan, add the bacon, chopped cabbage leaves, onion and garlic and fry until the onion is softened. Remove from the heat. Mix together the egg, cheese, parsley and salt and pepper to taste and stir into the cabbage mixture.

Place the cabbage 'shell' of large outside leaves in a casserole lined with foil and fill the shell with the fried mixture. Pour over the stock. Cover and cook in the oven for 1 hour. Uncover the casserole and cook for a further 30 minutes. To serve, lift the cabbage out, then remove the foil.

Cook's Tip

Fresh vine leaves can be used if they are first blanched in boiling water for 2 minutes, then drained and rinsed in cold water. Any stalks should be removed as these would make it difficult to fold the leaves into parcels.

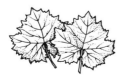

Cook's Tip

Try varying the ingredients of the stuffing by using lean minced beef or chicken dice instead of the bacon. You can omit the Parmesan cheese and use some concentrated tomato purée as a flavouring.

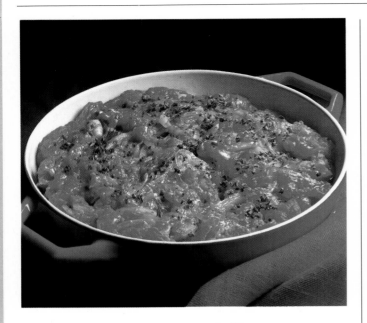

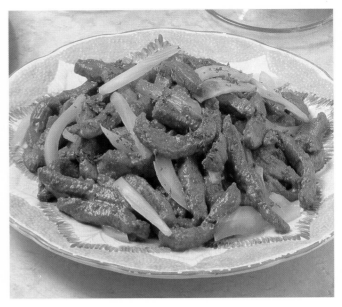

137 | Liver and Bacon Hotpot

Preparation time
15 minutes

Cooking time
1½ hours

Oven temperature
180°C, 350°F, gas 4

Serves 4

Calories
519 per portion

You will need
1 large onion, sliced
2 cooking apples, peeled, cored and sliced
150 g/5 oz mushrooms, sliced
200 g/7 oz unsmoked back bacon rashers, derinded
750 g/1 ½ lb lamb's liver, sliced
salt and pepper
½ x 400-g/14-oz can consommé
1 x 400-g/14-oz can tomatoes, drained and chopped
chopped parsley, to garnish

Spread one-third of the onion over the bottom of a casserole. Add one-third of the apple slices, then one-third of the mushrooms and bacon, then half the liver. Season well. Continue making layers in this way. Pour in the consommé and spread the tomatoes over the top.

Cover tightly and cook in the oven for 1½ hours. Serve garnished with chopped parsley.

138 | Stir-fried Liver and Fennel

Preparation time
15 minutes

Cooking time
12-15 minutes

Serves 6

Calories
214 per portion

You will need
750 g/1½ lb calves' liver, trimmed
1 tablespoon oil
1 large fennel bulb, finely sliced into thin strips
3 garlic cloves, chopped
3 tablespoons tomato purée
3 tablespoons red wine
salt and pepper
1 tablespoon chopped parsley

Cut the liver into 1 cm/1½ inch-wide strips.

Heat the oil in a heavy frying pan or a wok and add the fennel and garlic. Stir and cook for a few minutes over a medium to high heat. As soon as the fennel begins to colour slightly, add the liver and stir continuously. After 1 minute add the tomato purée and wine, bring to boiling point, simmer for 2 minutes, then remove from the heat. Add salt and pepper to taste and stir in the parsley.

Serve with rice or steamed potatoes and salad.

Cook's Tip

Both ox and pig's liver are slightly lower in calories than lamb's and cheaper. If you cut ox or pig's liver in slices and soak overnight in skimmed milk with a teaspoonful of bicarbonate of soda, it will be much improved.

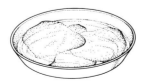

Cook's Tip

If you know your guests like liver, this way of cooking the finest variety is perfect for a dinner party. It has to be cooked just before serving but you can prepare everything in advance.

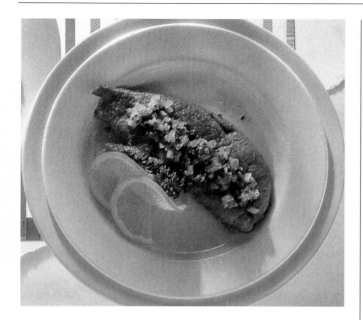

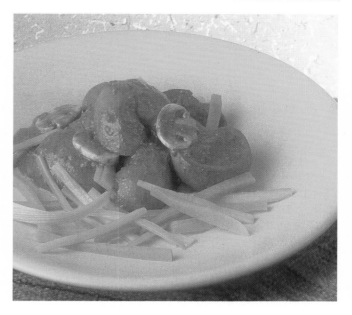

139 | Liver in Orange Sauce

Preparation time
10 minutes

Cooking time
8-10 minutes

Serves 4

Calories
264 per portion

You will need
4 thin slices lamb's liver, about 100 g/4 oz each
2 tablespoons seasoned flour for coating
15 g/½ oz butter
1 tablespoon olive oil
4 shallots, finely chopped
150 ml/¼ pint orange juice
1 teaspoon finely grated orange rind
salt and pepper
2 tablespoons chopped parsley

For the garnish
orange slices
parsley sprigs

Toss the liver in the seasoned flour, shaking off any excess. Heat the butter and oil in a large non-stick frying pan and fry two pieces of liver at a time for 2 minutes on each side, until browned on the outside and pale pink inside. Transfer to a warmed serving dish and keep warm.

Add the shallots to the pan and cook for 2 minutes, without browning. Lower the heat, add the orange juice and rind and boil for 2 minutes, stirring. Season with salt and pepper to taste and stir in the parsley. Spoon over the liver, garnish with orange slices and parsley and serve immediately.

Cook's Tip

Put the seasoned flour in a polythene bag, making sure it has no holes, add the slices of liver one at a time and toss until coated lightly. This way the flour will not be blown all over the kitchen.

140 | Sautéed Kidneys with Vegetable Julienne

Preparation time
20 minutes

Cooking time
20 minutes

Serves 6

Calories
167 per portion

You will need
12 lambs' kidneys, skinned, halved and cored
2 teaspoons seasoned flour
1 small onion, chopped
1 tablespoon olive oil
3 carrots, peeled and cut into julienne strips
2 leeks, cleaned and cut into julienne strips
100 g/4 oz button mushrooms, thinly sliced
150 ml/¼ pint beef stock
4 tablespoons dry sherry
salt and pepper

For the garnish
julienne strips of carrot, blanched
julienne strips of leek, blanched

Dust the lambs' kidneys very lightly with seasoned flour. Fry the onion gently in the oil for 3-4 minutes, add the kidneys and fry until sealed on all sides.

Add the strips of carrot and leek and the sliced mushrooms and fry together for 1 minute. Stir in the stock and sherry and bring to the boil; add salt and pepper to taste, and simmer gently until the kidneys are just tender (12-15 minutes).

Serve garnished with the blanched strips of carrot and leek.

Cook's Tip

Most supermarkets and chain stores sell kidneys ready prepared. If you buy them from a butcher they may still be covered with suet. Cut this away and remove the skin easily by nicking with the tip of a pointed knife.

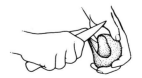

Poultry and Game

Provided that the fatty skin is removed, chicken is an ideal choice for a main course, being high in protein. Many of the recipes in this chapter feature chicken portions which are so easy to cook and can taste so good with fresh herbs, spices and citrus fruit. Turkey is almost equally versatile. A few special recipes for game have also been included, such as the delectable Wild Duck with Satsuma Sauce.

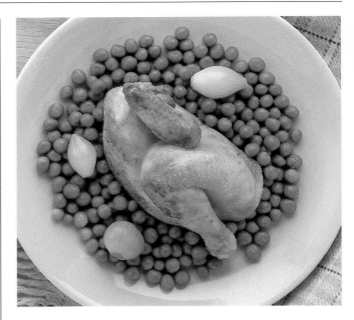

141 | Chicken and Leeks

Preparation time
20 minutes, plus standing

Cooking time
3-4 minutes

Serves 4

Calories
189 per portion

You will need
½ cucumber
salt
350 g/12 oz boneless chicken breasts, skinned
2 tablespoons oil
3 leeks, thinly sliced diagonally
4 garlic cloves, thinly sliced
1 tablespoon light soy sauce
1 tablespoon dry sherry
1 dried red chilli, crumbled
1 tablespoon chopped coriander
coriander leaves, to garnish

Peel the cucumber, cut in half and remove the seeds with a teaspoon. Cut the flesh into 2.5 cm/1 inch cubes, put in a colander and sprinkle with salt. Set aside for 20 minutes, rinse well and drain.

Cut the chicken into 2.5 cm/1 inch cubes. Heat the oil in a non-stick frying pan, add the leeks and garlic and cook briskly for 30 seconds. Add the soy sauce, sherry and chilli and cook for a further 30 seconds. Stir in the cucumber and cook for 30 seconds.

Transfer to a warmed serving dish, sprinkle with the chopped coriander, garnish with coriander leaves and serve immediately.

142 | Poussins with Peas

Preparation time
30 minutes

Cooking time
55 minutes

Serves 6

Calories
292 per portion

You will need
1 tablespoon olive oil
18 very small onions, shallots, or large spring onions
3 garlic cloves, very finely chopped
3 fresh poussins, about 350 g/ 12 oz each, halved down the backbone
175 ml/6 fl oz dry white wine
350 ml/12 fl oz hot water
salt and pepper
1 kg/2 ¼ lb peas, shelled weight

Heat the oil in a large heavy-based non-stick frying pan and fry the garlic and onions until light golden, then remove.

Fry the poussins, turning frequently until sealed and browned all over, then add the wine. As soon as it boils, add the water and salt and pepper to taste. Cover and simmer for 20 minutes, then uncover and simmer for another 20 minutes, adding the peas and onions about 8 minutes before cooking is completed.

Cook's Tip

Try eating Chinese dishes with chopsticks. Hold one stick firmly in the angle between your thumb and first finger, balancing it against the first joint of your third finger. The second stick is held between the top of your thumb and the inside of your forefinger and is pivoted to pick up pieces of food.

Cook's Tip

It may surprise you to know that frozen peas are much higher in fibre than fresh ones. Fibre is considered to be an excellent means of maintaining good health. It is only found in foods of vegetable origin.

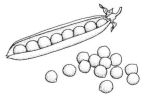

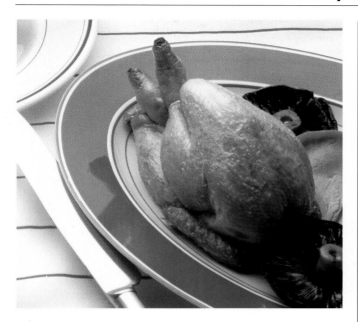

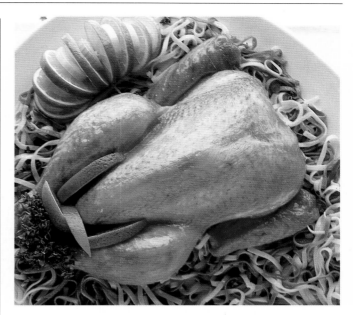

143 | *Braised Spring Chicken*

Preparation time
10 minutes

Cooking time
1 hour 5 minutes

Oven temperature
200°C, 400°F, gas 6

Serves 4

Calories
626 per portion

You will need
4 large flat mushrooms
2 teaspoons chopped fresh thyme
4 slices lean ham, without fat
2 spring chickens, prepared
salt and pepper
150 ml/¼ pint dry white wine

Cut off the mushroom stalks and place the mushrooms in the bottom of a large casserole. Sprinkle over the thyme. Lay the slices of ham over the mushrooms. Place the spring chickens on top. Add salt, pepper and the white wine.

Cover and cook in the oven for about 1 hour. Uncover and continue cooking for 5 minutes.

Cut each spring chicken in half and serve on a bed of mushrooms and ham.

144 | *Surprise Spring Chicken*

Preparation time
15 minutes, plus marinating

Cooking time
1½ hours

Oven temperature
190°C, 375°F, gas 5

Serves 4

Calories
351 per portion

You will need
2 limes
1 small onion, cut into 8 slices
1 x 1-1.25 kg/2¼-2¾ lb spring chicken, prepared
25 g/1 oz raisins
2 tablespoons olive oil
pinch of chilli powder
sea salt

For the garnish
lime slices
onion slices

Slash one lime almost through in 8 places and insert an onion slice in each cut. Place inside the chicken cavity with the raisins.

Squeeze the juice from the remaining lime and mix with the oil, chilli powder and salt to taste. Pour over the chicken and leave to marinate for 1 hour.

Truss the chicken securely and place in a roasting pan. Cook in the oven for 1½ hours, basting twice, or until the juices run clear yellow.

Serve the chicken with its juices on a bed of noodles. Garnish with lime and onion slices.

Cook's Tip

If fresh thyme is not available, replace with half the quantity of dried thyme. This herb retains its aroma for quite a long time after drying but fresh thyme does, of course, have a better flavour.

Cook's Tip

Always remove the giblets from a fresh chicken as soon as possible and place an onion in the cavity to keep it sweet until it is cooked. Use the giblets immediately to make stock which can be frozen, if liked.

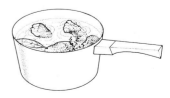

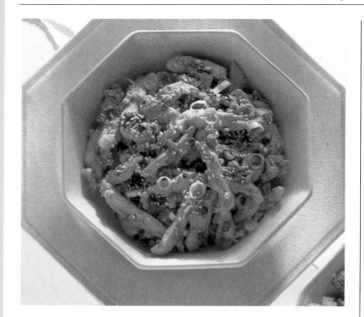

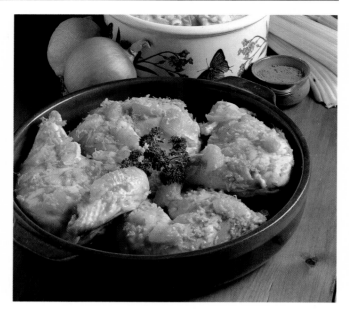

145 | *Chicken with Sesame Seeds*

Preparation time
15 minutes, plus standing

Cooking time
5 minutes

Serves 4

Calories
208 per portion

You will need
350 g/12 oz boneless chicken
  breasts
1 egg white
½ teaspoon salt
2 teaspoons cornflour
2 tablespoons white sesame
  seeds
2 tablespoons oil
1 tablespoon dark soy sauce
1 tablespoon wine vinegar
½ teaspoon chilli bean sauce
½ teaspoon sesame oil
½ teaspoon roasted Szechuan
  peppercorns
4 spring onions, chopped

Cut the chicken into 7.5 cm/3 inch long shreds. Combine the egg white, salt and cornflour, toss in the chicken and mix thoroughly. Leave to stand for 15 minutes.

Cook the sesame seeds in a large non-stick frying pan until they are golden brown. Remove from the pan and set aside.

Heat the oil in the pan, add the chicken and stir-fry briskly for 1 minute. Remove with a slotted spoon. Add the soy sauce, vinegar, chilli bean sauce, sesame oil and peppercorns to the pan and bring to the boil. Add the chicken and spring onions and cook for 2 minutes. Sprinkle with the sesame seeds and serve immediately.

146 | *Citrus Chicken*

Preparation time
10 minutes

Cooking time
1 hour

Oven temperature
190°C, 375°F, gas 5

Serves 4

Calories
220 per portion

You will need
4 chicken quarters, about 225 g/
  8 oz each, skinned
salt and pepper
ground cinnamon
2 large lemons or limes
2 large oranges
15 g/½ oz butter
parsley sprigs, to garnish

Rub the chicken quarters with salt and pepper and a little cinnamon. Place in a lightly oiled casserole.

Squeeze the juice from one of the lemons or limes and pour over the chicken. Grate the rind from one of the oranges. Peel the remaining lemon or lime and both oranges and chop the flesh. Mix the flesh with the grated orange rind and pour over the chicken. Dot the chicken and fruit with the butter.

Cover tightly and cook in the oven for 1 hour, or until tender. Garnish with parsley.

Cook's Tip

There are considerable regional variations in Chinese cooking depending on the climate and what crops are grown. Szechuan province, on the Tibetan border, is renowned for its fiery dishes such as this one.

Cook's Tip

Limes are slightly sweeter and have a more subtle flavour than lemons. You can tell a fresh lime by its dark, glossy, tight skin. Both the rind and juice of a lime can be used in the same way as a lemon.

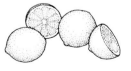

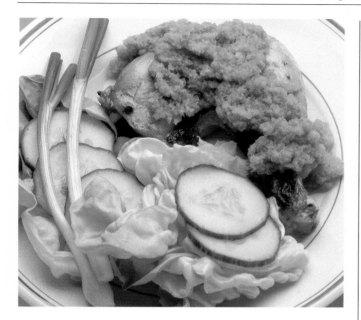

147 | *West Indian Chicken*

Preparation time
20 minutes, plus
marinating

Cooking time
25 minutes

Serves 4

Calories
215 per portion

You will need
4 chicken portions, about 175 g/
  6 oz each, skinned
1 teaspoon curry powder, or to
  taste
1 teaspoon ground ginger
1 x 225-g/8-oz can pineapple
  chunks in natural juice
1 green pepper, seeded and
  chopped
salt and pepper

Score the flesh of the chicken portions with a sharp knife. Mix the curry powder and ginger together and rub into the chicken flesh. Place the chicken portions in a shallow dish and pour over the pineapple juice from the can. Leave to marinate for 2 hours.

Put the chicken portions under a hot grill and cook for about 20 minutes until tender, turning frequently and using the marinade to baste and prevent burning.

Put the pineapple chunks, remaining marinade and chopped pepper into a blender and liquidize until smooth. Pour the purée into a pan and heat through. Taste and adjust the seasoning.

Arrange the grilled chicken portions on a warmed serving dish and pour the sauce over or serve it separately. Serve with a green salad.

Cook's Tip

Although the pineapple is native to the Guyanas and Brazil, it has been grown in Jamaica for many years. Fresh fruit is used there to make this chicken dish but the canned variety involves less preparation.

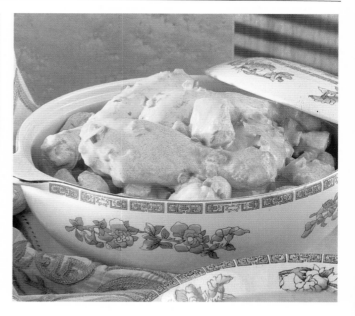

148 | *Spiced Chicken*

Preparation time
15 minutes, plus
marinating

Cooking time
1¼ hours

Serves 6

Calories
240 per portion

You will need
1 teaspoon ground cinnamon
6 chicken drumsticks, skinned
3 chicken breasts, about 175 g/
  6 oz each, boned and skinned
300 ml/½ pint natural low-fat
  yogurt
1 tablespoon oil
2 large onions, chopped
2 fresh green chillis, seeded and
  chopped
1 teaspoon cumin seeds
1 garlic clove, chopped
1 tablespoon sweet paprika
2 tablespoons chicken stock
½ teaspoon finely grated lemon
  rind
1 red pepper, seeded and
  chopped
1 tablespoon cornflour
salt and pepper

Rub the cinnamon into the chicken meat, combine with the yogurt and marinate for about 30 minutes.

Heat the oil in a flameproof casserole and lightly fry the onions, chillis, cumin and garlic. Stir in the paprika.

Strain the chicken meat, reserving the yogurt. Add the chicken to the casserole, stir well to coat and then add the stock, lemon rind, red pepper and half of the reserved yogurt. Cover and simmer slowly for about 1 hour.

A few minutes before serving, combine the cornflour with the remaining yogurt and stir it into the casserole, bring to the boil and simmer for 1-2 minutes. Taste and add salt and pepper. Serve with rice.

Cook's Tip

If you like spicy foods, try keeping a dried chilli in the storage jar with the rice. It will impart its distinctive flavour in the same way as a vanilla pod kept in a jar of sugar.

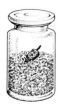

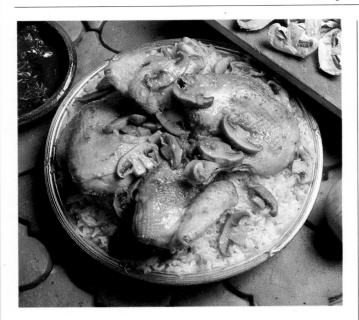

149 | Chicken with Herbs and Rice

Preparation time
20 minutes

Cooking time
1¼ hours

Serves 4

Calories
331 per portion

You will need
2 tablespoons oil
1 onion, chopped
2 garlic cloves, chopped
4 chicken portions
100 g/4 oz mushrooms, sliced
150 ml/¼ pint chicken stock
150 ml/¼ pint dry cider
2 teaspoons chopped fresh mixed
  herbs
salt and pepper
100 g/4 oz long-grain rice
pinch of powdered saffron

Heat the oil in a non-stick frying pan. Fry the onion and garlic with the chicken portions until golden. Add the mushrooms, stock, cider, herbs and salt and pepper. Cover and simmer gently for 1 hour.

Meanwhile cook the rice (see Cook's Tip). Stir the saffron into the cooked rice.

To serve, arrange the rice on a warmed serving dish, put the chicken pieces and vegetables on top.

150 | Cashew Chicken

Preparation time
20 minutes

Cooking time
3-4 minutes

Serves 4

Calories
208 per portion

You will need
350 g/12 oz boneless chicken
  breasts, skinned
1 egg white
2 tablespoons dry sherry
2 teaspoons cornflour
2 tablespoons oil
4 spring onions, chopped
2 garlic cloves, thinly sliced
1 x 2.5 cm/1 inch piece root
  ginger, finely chopped
1 tablespoon light soy sauce
50 g/2 oz unsalted cashew nuts

Cut the chicken into 1 cm/½ inch cubes. Combine the egg white, half the sherry and the cornflour, add the chicken and toss well until evenly coated.

Heat the oil in a large non-stick frying pan, add the spring onions, garlic and ginger and stir fry for 30 seconds. Add the chicken and cook for 2 minutes. Pour in the remaining sherry and the soy sauce and stir well. Add the cashew nuts and cook for a further 30 seconds. Serve immediately.

Cook's Tip

To cook the rice, put it in a saucepan with 300 ml/½ pint cold water. Bring to the boil, then cover and simmer for 35-40 minutes, until the water has been absorbed and the rice is tender.

Cook's Tip

A wok is traditionally used for this type of rapid cooking. There are two basic designs: one with a short, round handle on either side and one with a long handle. The former is better for steaming.

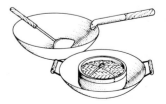

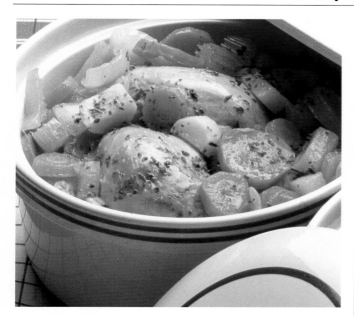

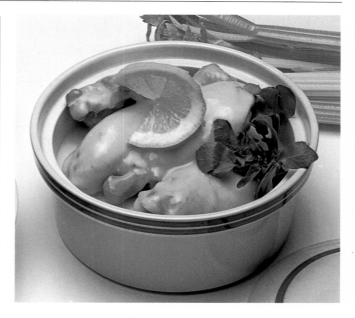

151 | Chicken and Vegetable Casserole

Preparation time
25 minutes

Cooking time
1½ hours

Oven temperature
180°C, 350°F, gas 4

Serves 4

Calories
265 per portion

You will need
1 onion, roughly chopped
3-4 celery sticks, roughly chopped
4 carrots, peeled and roughly chopped
4 turnips, peeled and roughly chopped
1 small swede, peeled and roughly chopped
4 chicken portions, about 175 g/ 6 oz each, skinned
1 bay leaf
1 bouquet garni (see Recipe 109)
300 ml/½ pint chicken stock
salt and pepper

Put half of the vegetables in a casserole. Put the chicken portions on top and cover with the remaining vegetables. Add the bay leaf, bouquet garni, stock, salt and pepper to taste. If using a flameproof casserole, bring to the boil on top of the cooker and skim.

Cover and cook in the oven for about 1½ hours. Skim off any fat and serve.

152 | Chicken in Lemon Sauce

Preparation time
20 minutes

Cooking time
1 hour 10 minutes

Oven temperature
190°C, 375°F, gas 5

Serves 4

Calories
228 per portion

You will need
4 chicken portions, about 175 g/ 6 oz each, skinned
grated rind and juice of 1 lemon
1 small onion, chopped
1 celery stick, chopped
few thyme sprigs
salt and pepper
300 ml/½ pint chicken stock
15 g/½ oz cornflour

For the garnish
watercress
lemon twists

Put the chicken in a 1.75 litre/3 pint casserole. Add the lemon rind and juice, onion, celery, thyme, salt and pepper to taste, and the stock. Cover and cook in the oven for 1 hour, or until the chicken is tender.

Transfer the chicken to a serving dish and keep hot. Strain the stock.

Mix the cornflour to a smooth paste with a little of the stock. Then combine with the remaining stock and cook over a low heat, stirring constantly, until thickened. Check the seasoning and pour the sauce over the chicken. Garnish with watercress and lemon.

Cook's Tip

If you cook this casserole the day before, it can be put in the refrigerator overnight and reheated for 30 minutes before serving. The fat is easier to remove when it is cold.

Cook's Tip

Using cornflour to thicken sauces rather than a roux made of butter and flour cuts the calories. Clear sauces should be thickened with potato flour as this will not cloud the sauce.

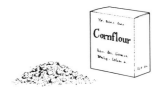

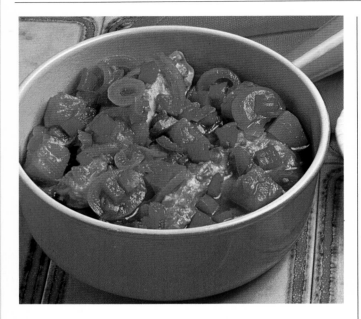

153 | Chicken in Sweet and Sour Sauce

Preparation time
20 minutes

Cooking time
1 hour

Oven temperature
190°C, 375°F, gas 5

Serves 4

Calories
264 per portion

You will need
4 chicken portions, about 175 g/
   6 oz each, skinned
1 green pepper, seeded and
   chopped
1 red pepper, seeded and
   chopped
1 onion, sliced
1 x 225-g/8-oz can pineapple
   pieces in natural juice, drained
1 tablespoon soy sauce
1 tablespoon vinegar
1 x 225-g/8-oz can tomatoes
150 ml/¼ pint water
1 teaspoon clear honey
salt

Put the chicken portions in a 1.75 litre/3 pint casserole and cook, uncovered, in the oven for 15 minutes.

Put the remaining ingredients, with salt to taste, in a saucepan. Bring to the boil, stirring, cover and simmer for 20 minutes. Pour the sauce over the chicken and return to the oven for a further 30 minutes, or until the chicken is tender, basting occasionally with the sauce. Serve with green vegetables.

Cook's Tip

The natural sweetness of pineapple makes it a perfect fruit to use in sweet'n'sour dishes. It combines particularly well with chicken and the other ingredients in this appetizing casserole.

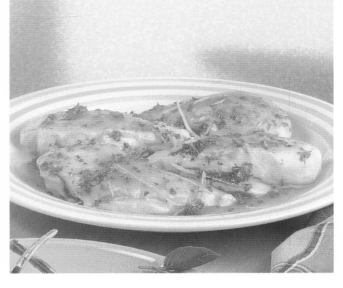

154 | Lemon Chicken

Preparation time
25 minutes

Cooking time
30-35 minutes

Serves 4

Calories
220 per portion

You will need
1 lemon, very thinly peeled, rind
   reserved
1 small onion, thinly sliced
1 tablespoon olive oil
4 chicken breasts, about 150 g/
   5 oz each, skinned and boned
2 tablespoons chopped parsley
300 ml/½ pint chicken stock
salt and pepper
2 teaspoons cornflour
1 tablespoon water

Cut the lemon rind into matchstick strips. Halve the lemon and squeeze out the juice.

Fry the onion gently in the oil for 3-4 minutes, then add the chicken breasts and fry until lightly browned on all sides. Add the parsley, stock, salt and pepper to taste and lemon juice; cover the pan and simmer gently for 20 minutes. Remove the chicken breasts to a warmed serving dish, and keep hot.

Blend the cornflour and water to a smooth paste; stir in the hot cooking liquid, and then return to the pan. Stir over a gentle heat until thickened. Add the strips of lemon rind to the sauce and spoon evenly over the chicken.

Cook's Tip

Lemons can be stored for some weeks in the crisper drawer of a refrigerator, so buy in quantity during their peak season. The smooth-skinned variety are juicier while lemons with a rougher skin are easier to grate.

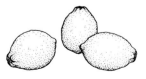

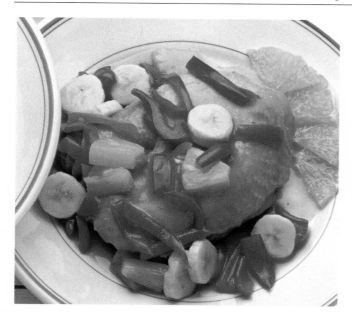

155 | Caribbean Chicken

Preparation time
15 minutes

Cooking time
1 hour

Oven temperature
220°C, 425°F, gas 7

Serves 4

Calories
284 per portion

You will need
4 chicken portions, about 175 g/
  6 oz each, skinned
1 large red pepper, seeded and
  chopped
1 teaspoon curry powder
250 ml/8 fl oz chicken stock
salt and pepper
4 pineapple rings, fresh or canned
  in natural juice
1 banana
1 orange, peeled and sliced, to
  garnish

Put the chicken portions in a casserole with the chopped pepper and curry powder. Pour over the stock and add salt and pepper to taste. Cover and cook in the oven for 50 minutes.

Chop the pineapple rings and banana and add to the casserole. Cook for a further 10 minutes, or until the chicken is tender.

Garnish the casserole with the orange slices.

156 | Spicy Chicken and Peanuts

Preparation time
20 minutes

Cooking time
5 minutes

Serves 4

Calories
272 per portion

You will need
50 g/2 oz unsalted peanuts
350 g/12 oz boneless chicken
  breasts, skinned
2 tablespoons oil
1 dried red chilli
1 tablespoon dry sherry
1 tablespoon dark soy sauce
pinch of sugar
1 garlic clove, crushed
2 spring onions, chopped
1 x 2.5 cm/1 inch piece root
  ginger, finely chopped
1 teaspoon wine vinegar
2 teaspoons sesame oil
red chilli flowers, to garnish (see
  Cook's Tip)

Immerse the peanuts in a bowl of boiling water for about 2 minutes. Drain well, remove the skins and put on absorbent kitchen paper to dry thoroughly. Cut the chicken into 2.5 cm/1 inch cubes.

Heat the oil in a large non-stick frying pan. Crumble in the chilli, add the chicken and peanuts and stir-fry for 1 minute; remove from the pan. Add the sherry, soy sauce, sugar, garlic, spring onions, ginger and vinegar to the pan. Bring to the boil, then simmer for 30 seconds. Return the chicken, chilli and peanuts to the pan and cook for 2 minutes. Sprinkle over the sesame oil.

Pile into a warmed serving dish, garnish with red chilli flowers and serve immediately.

Cook's Tip

Caribbean food is usually highly spiced. Curry powder is often made at home with freshly ground spices such as coriander seeds, turmeric, fenugreek, ginger, black pepper, cardamom and cinnamon.

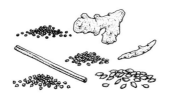

Cook's Tip

To make chilli flowers, shred the chilli lengthways leaving 1 cm/½ inch attached at the stem end. Put in a bowl of iced water for about 1 hour or until it opens.

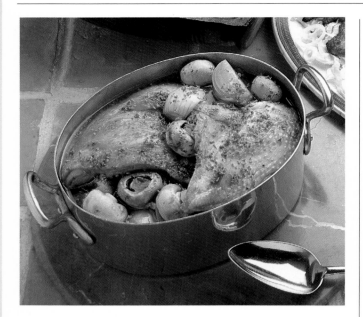

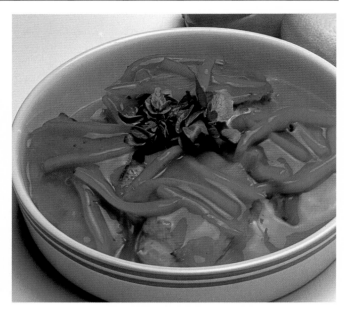

157 | Slimmer's Coq au Vin

Preparation time
20 minutes, plus
marinating

Cooking time
1 hour 10 minutes

Oven temperature
220°C, 425°F, gas 7

Serves 4

Calories
259 per portion

You will need
4 chicken portions, about 175 g/
   6 oz each, skinned
2 tablespoons brandy
225 g/8 oz baby onions, peeled
900 ml/1½ pints chicken stock
225 g/8 oz button mushrooms,
   wiped and trimmed
chopped fresh parsley, to garnish

For the marinade
1 garlic clove, crushed
150 ml/¼ pint red wine vinegar
150 ml/¼ pint red wine
1 tablespoon Worcestershire
   sauce
salt and pepper

Combine all the marinade ingredients. Put the chicken in a large shallow bowl and pour over the marinade. Set aside in a cool place for at least 3 hours.

Remove the chicken portions from the marinade (reserving the marinade), and brown briefly under the grill. Transfer the chicken to a casserole. Pour the brandy over the chicken and ignite. When the flames die, add the onions and stock. Cover and cook in the oven for 50 minutes. Add the mushrooms and cook for 10 minutes, or until the chicken is tender and the juices run clear.

Meanwhile, pour the marinade into a saucepan and boil rapidly, uncovered, until reduced in volume by half. Stir into the casserole and garnish with the parsley.

158 | Italian Chicken

Preparation time
25 minutes

Cooking time
1 hour

Oven temperature
180°C, 350°F, gas 4

Serves 4

Calories
204 per portion

You will need
4 chicken breasts, skinned and
   boned
50 g/2 oz lean ham, cut into 4
   pieces
150 ml/¼ pint chicken stock
1 red pepper, seeded and sliced
watercress sprigs, to garnish

For the stuffing
40 g/1½ oz wholemeal
   breadcrumbs
25 g/1 oz Parmesan cheese,
   grated
1 small onion, finely chopped
2 teaspoons chopped parsley
1 tablespoon dry sherry
salt and pepper

Mix together the stuffing ingredients, with salt and pepper to taste, and press to the underside of the chicken breasts. Place a piece of ham over the top. Arrange the chicken in a casserole, pour over the stock and add the red pepper.

Cover and cook in the oven for 1 hour, or until the chicken is cooked, basting occasionally with the liquid. Garnish with watercress.

Cook's Tip

Mushrooms are best stored in the refrigerator in a paper or fabric bag. If you have bought them loose, avoid leaving them in a plastic bag. It is not necessary to peel them unless the skins are very soiled by their growing medium.

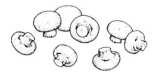

Cook's Tip

Freshly grated Parmesan would always be used by any Italian who prided themselves on their cooking. Most large supermarkets now sell small blocks of Parmesan as well as drums of the grated kind.

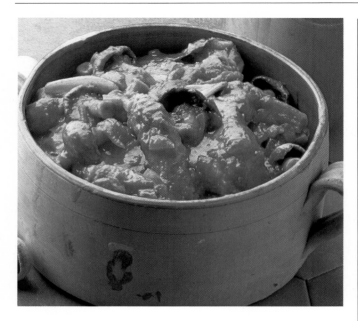

159 | *Poulet Chasseur*

Preparation time
25 minutes

Cooking time
1½ hours

Serves 6

Calories
306 per portion

You will need
2 tablespoons oil
1 x 1.75 kg/4 lb chicken, cut into
  serving pieces
100 g/4 oz baby onions
250 g/8 oz shallots, chopped
150 ml/¼ pint dry vermouth
1 bouquet garni (see Recipe 109)
1 bay leaf
salt and pepper
1 x 400-g/14-oz can tomatoes
225 g/8 oz button mushrooms
1 tablespoon tomato purée

Heat the oil in a non-stick frying pan, add the chicken pieces and fry until browned on all sides. Remove from the pan. Add the onions and shallots to the pan and cook for 5 minutes.

Remove the pan from the heat, add the vermouth and ignite. When the flames have died down, return the chicken to the pan and add the bouquet garni, bay leaf, and salt and pepper to taste. Add the tomatoes with their juice, bring to the boil, cover and simmer for 1 hour.

Add the mushrooms and tomato purée and cook, uncovered, for 20-30 minutes, until the sauce is reduced and thickened. Serve immediately.

Cook's Tip

For authenticity, use a French vermouth. This is drier than the Italian. If you warm the vermouth before igniting it, it will be more effective. Choose the least expensive type of vermouth for cooking.

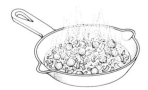

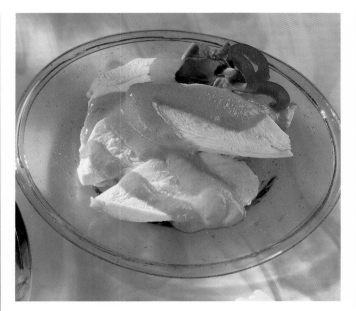

160 | *Pimento Chicken*

Preparation time
1 hour

Cooking time
2¼ hours

Serves 8

Calories
315 per portion

You will need
1 x 1.75 kg/4 lb oven-ready
  chicken
1 onion, quartered
1 carrot, sliced
2 celery sticks, sliced
4 juniper berries, crushed
1 bay leaf
4-6 stalks parsley
salt
6 peppercorns, lightly crushed

For the sauce
225 g/8 oz canned pimentos,
  drained, rinsed and chopped
1 tablespoon tomato purée
2 tablespoons mango chutney
200 ml/7 fl oz low-fat yogurt
freshly ground black pepper

Put the chicken, vegetables, juniper berries, bay leaf, parsley, salt and peppercorns into a saucepan. Cover with water. Bring to the boil, cover the saucepan and simmer for 1½-2 hours, or until the chicken is tender. Leave the chicken to cool in the stock. Lift out the chicken, drain and dry it. (Reserve the stock, discarding the bay leaf.) Skin the chicken and slice the meat from the bones.

To make the sauce, put the pimentos, 2 tablespoons of the reserved chicken stock, tomato purée and chutney into a saucepan and bring to the boil. Liquidize in a blender and set aside to cool. Blend the cooled pimento mixture with the yogurt and season with salt and pepper.

Arrange the chicken on a dish and cover with the sauce. Serve with pepper rings, tomato and watercress.

Cook's Tip

This is an excellent way of serving chicken at a summer lunch party as it can be prepared in advance. Serve with a choice of colourful salads to complement the garnish.

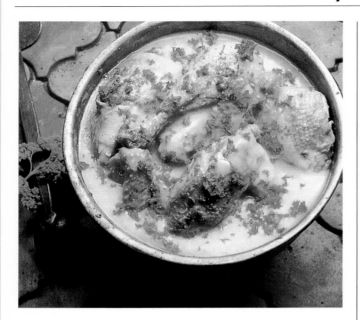

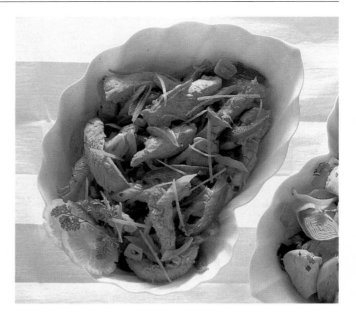

161 | Chicken with Yogurt

Preparation time
20 minutes

Cooking time
1 hour 10 minutes

Serves 4

Calories
491 per portion

You will need
1 x 1.5 kg/3 lb chicken
1 onion, chopped
1 garlic clove, crushed
½ green pepper, seeded and
  chopped
2 tablespoons oil
25 g/1 oz cornflour
600 ml/1 pint chicken stock
salt and pepper
300 ml/½ pint natural low-fat
  yogurt

For the garnish
chopped fresh chives or parsley

Cut the chicken into portions. Heat the oil in a flameproof casserole or saucepan. Add the chicken pieces, onion, green pepper and garlic and fry the chicken until lightly browned on all sides.

Mix the cornflour to a smooth paste with a little of the stock. Then combine with the remaining stock and cook over a low heat, stirring constantly until thickened. Pour over the chicken, cover the casserole or saucepan and simmer for 30 minutes. Stir in the yogurt and continue cooking gently for 30 minutes. Adjust the seasoning to taste before serving. Sprinkle lightly with chopped chives or parsley.

Cook's Tip

A garlic press is the easiest way of crushing the cloves. Unfortunately, the smell of garlic lingers however carefully you clean the garlic press so keep it in a polythene bag. Remove stubborn threads of garlic with a pin.

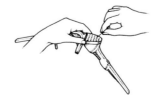

162 | Chicken with Ginger

Preparation time
20 minutes, plus
marinating

Cooking time
4-5 minutes

Serves 4

Calories
182 per portion

You will need
350 g/12 oz boneless chicken
  breasts, skinned
1 tablespoon dry sherry
4 spring onions, chopped
1 x 2.5 cm/1 inch piece fresh root
  ginger, finely chopped
2 tablespoons oil
1-2 garlic cloves, thinly sliced
2 celery sticks, sliced diagonally
1 small green pepper, seeded and
  sliced
2 tablespoons light soy sauce
juice of ½ lemon
shredded rind of 2 lemons
¼ teaspoon chilli powder

For the garnish
lemon slices
parsley sprigs

Cut the chicken into 7.5 cm/3 inch strips. Combine the sherry, spring onions and ginger, add the chicken and toss well to coat, then set aside for 15 minutes.

Heat the oil in a large non-stick frying pan or wok. Add the garlic, celery and green pepper and stir-fry for 1 minute. Add the chicken and marinade and cook for 2 minutes. Stir in the soy sauce, lemon juice and rind and chilli powder and cook for a further 1 minute.

Pile into a warmed serving dish, garnish with lemon slices and parsley sprigs and serve immediately.

Cook's Tip

If you cannot find any fresh root ginger locally, use the dried kind. The best quality ginger comes from Jamaica and is usually available in markets supplying ethnic communities, as well as in some large supermarkets.

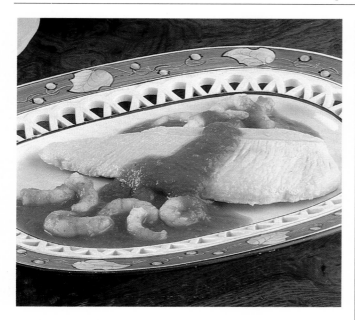

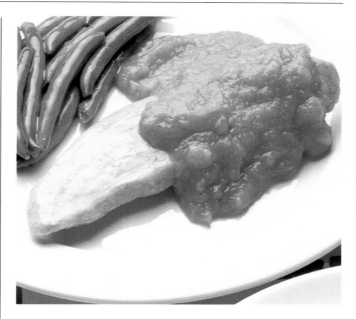

163 | Turkey Fillets with Piquant Prawn Sauce

Preparation time
25 minutes

Cooking time
30-35 minutes

Oven temperature
190-200°C, 375-400°F, gas 5-6

Serves 6

Calories
243 per portion

You will need
3 red peppers, seeded and chopped
1 chilli, seeded and cut into 6
3 garlic cloves, chopped
3 tomatoes, peeled, seeded and chopped
1 aubergine, finely chopped
salt and pepper
6 turkey fillets, about 175 g/6 oz each
1 tablespoon olive oil
1 tablespoon vinegar
1 teaspoon anchovy essence
175 g/6 oz peeled, cooked prawns

Put all the chopped vegetables in a bowl, sprinkle with salt and pepper, and mix well. Spread the mixture over a sheet of foil large enough to lay the turkey fillets on side by side. Put the fillets on top of the vegetables and paint with a little of the oil. Cover loosely with more foil and seal completely. Cook on a baking sheet in the preheated oven (the oven temperature depending on the thickness of the fillets), for 25-30 minutes. Remove the fillets to a warmed serving dish.

Heat the remaining oil in a saucepan and rub the cooked vegetables through a sieve on to it. Bring to the boil and add the vinegar, anchovy essence and prawns, adjust the seasoning and cook for 3-5 minutes. Spoon the sauce over the fillets.

Cook's Tip

Penne – the pasta that is shaped like a quill – or plain rice, mixed with a little diced cucumber, make good accompaniments to the turkey fillets with the piquant sauce.

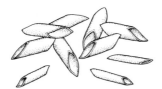

164 | Gingered Turkey

Preparation time
10 minutes, plus soaking

Cooking time
10 minutes

Serves 4

Calories
225 per portion

You will need
225 g/8 oz dried apricots
1-2 teaspoons ground ginger
4 turkey fillets, about 100 g/4 oz each

Put the apricots in a bowl. Just cover with water and add the ground ginger. Leave to soak overnight.

Next day, put the turkey fillets on the rack of a grill pan and spoon over a little of the apricot soaking liquid. Put under a hot grill for about 10 minutes, turning once. If necessary, spoon over more apricot liquid.

Meanwhile, simmer the apricots in the rest of the soaking liquid for about 10 minutes. Pour the cooked apricots into a blender and liquidize until smooth.

Arrange the cooked turkey fillets on a warmed serving dish and pour the apricot sauce over. Serve with green beans.

Cook's Tip

Dried apricots are one of the best sources of fibre. None of this is lost by liquidizing the fruit. They give a delicious flavour to the turkey fillets which can be a little bland.

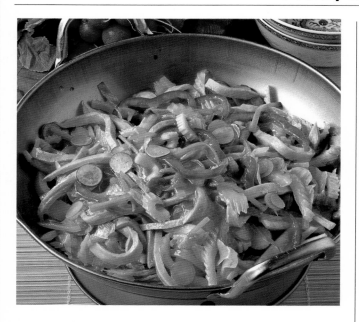

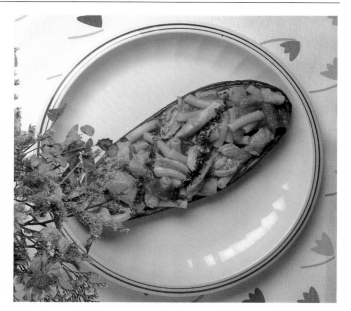

165 | *Sweet-sour Chinese Turkey*

Preparation time
15 minutes, plus
marinating

Cooking time
15-20 minutes

Serves 4

Calories
180 per portion

You will need
450 g/1 lb turkey breast
2 tablespoons lemon juice
5 tablespoons orange juice
4-5 celery sticks
2 sharon fruit or firm tomatoes
8-10 radishes
½ Chinese cabbage
1 large green pepper, seeded
2 tablespoons oil
150 ml/¼ pint chicken stock
1½ teaspoons cornflour
1 tablespoon soy sauce
1 tablespoon clear honey

Cut the turkey breast into thin strips. Marinate in the lemon and orange juice for 30 minutes. Cut the celery, sharon fruit or tomatoes, radishes and Chinese cabbage into small neat pieces. Heat the oil in a large non-stick frying pan. Drain the turkey and reserve the marinade. Fry the turkey in the oil until nearly tender. Add the vegetables and sharon fruit or tomatoes and heat for 2-3 minutes only. Blend the chicken stock with the marinade and the cornflour. Add the soy sauce and sugar. Pour over the ingredients in the pan and stir until thickened.

166 | *Turkey-stuffed Aubergines*

Preparation time
15 minutes, plus
draining

Cooking time
35 minutes

Oven temperature
200°C, 400°F, gas 6

Serves 4

Calories
194 per portion

You will need
2 large aubergines
lemon juice
salt and pepper
100 g/4 oz macaroni, cooked
350 g/12 oz cooked turkey meat,
    cut into chunks
300 ml/½ pint tomato juice
1 teaspoon ground coriander
parsley sprigs, to garnish

Cut each aubergine in half and sprinkle with lemon juice and salt. Leave to drain for at least 30 minutes.

Put each half on a piece of foil large enough to enclose it completely. Wrap the aubergine halves and cook in the oven for about 30 minutes.

Meanwhile, gently heat the macaroni and turkey meat in the tomato juice, coriander and salt and pepper to taste.

When the aubergines are tender, unwrap and carefully scoop out the flesh. Mix with the macaroni and turkey pieces and pile back into the aubergine shells. Return to the oven to heat through for 5 minutes. Serve immediately, sprinkled with parsley.

Cook's Tip

Sharon fruit is a variety of persimmon which can be eaten like an apple. The skin is edible or the fruit can be peeled. It is often candied.

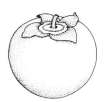

Cook's Tip

This is an appetizing way of using turkey leftovers. Turkey portions are easily available and some delicatessens and food shops also sell cooked turkey pieces. Remember to remove all the skin.

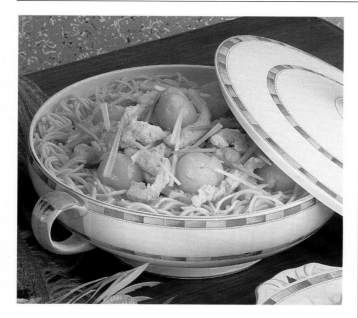

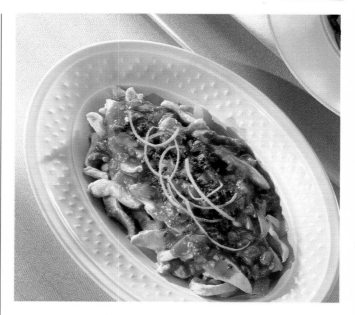

167 | Sesame Turkey with Ginger and Lychees

Preparation time
25 minutes

Cooking time
15-20 minutes

Serves 4

Calories
288 per portion

You will need
450 g/1 lb turkey fillets, cut into
  thin strips
1 egg, beaten
3 tablespoons sesame seeds
3 tablespoons olive oil
1 small onion, finely chopped
1 garlic clove, finely chopped
slice of fresh root ginger, 1 cm/
  ½ inch thick, finely chopped
2 tablespoons unsweetened
  pineapple juice
4 tablespoons chicken stock
12 fresh lychees, shelled
1 tablespoon lime juice
salt and pepper
julienne strips of spring onion, to
  garnish

Dip the strips of turkey into beaten egg, shaking off the excess, and coat lightly in sesame seeds.

Heat the olive oil in a shallow pan; add the onion and garlic and fry for 2-3 minutes. Add the ginger and the strips of turkey and fry until the turkey is evenly coloured. Pour over the pineapple juice and stock and simmer for 5 minutes, covered. Add the lychees and lime juice and season well to taste. Stir well, then simmer, covered for a further 4-5 minutes.

Serve, garnished with spring onion strips, on a bed of Chinese noodles.

Cook's Tip

Scrape away the outer skin of the fresh ginger before using. The stones can be removed from the lychees before adding to the casserole but do this in a dish so that none of the fragrant juice is wasted.

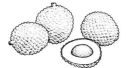

168 | Turkey with Walnuts

Preparation time
25 minutes

Cooking time
8-10 minutes

Serves 4

Calories
152 per portion

You will need
1 tablespoon oil
1 onion, finely chopped
1 garlic clove, crushed
1 turkey breast, skinned, sliced
  and cut into small slivers
grated rind and juice of 1 orange
25 g/1 oz walnuts, chopped
1 tablespoon soy sauce
2 teaspoons cornflour, blended
  with 4 tablespoons water
1 teaspoon clear honey
1 tablespoon finely chopped
  parsley
pepper
orange rind, shredded, to garnish

Heat the oil in a non-stick frying pan, add the onion and fry, stirring for 2 minutes. Stir in the garlic and push the mixture to one side of the pan. Tilt the pan to let the juices run out over the base. Add the turkey slivers and stir-fry for about 2 minutes. Remove with a slotted spoon and keep warm in a warmed serving dish.

Add the orange rind and juice, walnuts, soy sauce, blended cornflour, sugar and parsley to the pan. Bring to the boil, stirring, then simmer until thickened. Add pepper to taste and pour over the turkey. Garnish with orange rind.

Cook's Tip

Walnuts do not keep well as their oil tends to go rancid. They should therefore be bought in small quantities and used as soon as possible. When they are really fresh, the skin enclosing the kernel can easily be removed.

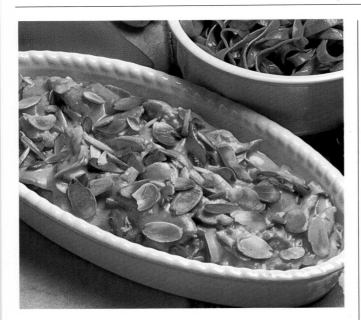

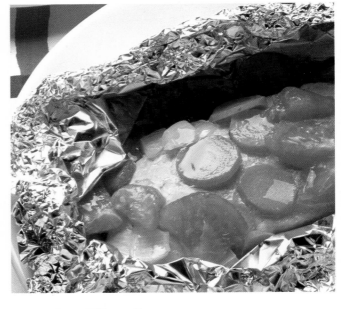

169 | *Turkey Sicilian-style*

Preparation time
20 minutes

Cooking time
30 minutes

Serves 4

Calories
209 per portion

You will need
25 g/1 oz butter
1 onion, sliced
75 g/3 oz button mushrooms, sliced
25 g/1 oz plain wholemeal flour
½ teaspoon ground ginger
½ teaspoon grated nutmeg
150 ml/¼ pint chicken stock
150 ml/¼ pint skimmed milk
350 g/12 oz cooked turkey meat, chopped
salt and pepper
15 g/½ oz flaked almonds, toasted

Melt the butter in a large saucepan, add the onion and mushrooms and fry gently for 5 minutes, or until soft. Add the flour, ginger and nutmeg. Cook for 1 minute. Gradually blend in the stock and milk. Bring to the boil, stirring, then add the turkey and salt and pepper to taste. Cover and simmer for 20 minutes.

Pile the mixture into a warmed serving dish and sprinkle with the toasted almonds. Serve with a small portion of noodles and salad.

170 | *Turkey Portugaise*

Preparation time
15 minutes

Cooking time
20 minutes

Oven temperature
220°C, 425°F, gas 7

Serves 4

Calories
131 per portion

You will need
4 turkey fillets, about 100 g/4 oz each
1 garlic clove, crushed
2 tomatoes, roughly chopped
1 carrot, peeled and very thinly sliced
25 g/1 oz onion, chopped
salt and pepper

Put each turkey fillet on a piece of foil large enough to cover it. Spread a little crushed garlic on each one. Divide the tomato, carrot and onion between the fillets. Sprinkle with salt and pepper. Wrap the fillets completely in foil and cook in the oven for about 20 minutes until tender.

Cook's Tip

With such a large variety of fresh pasta now available, it is easy to experiment with different kinds. Children will like the new pasta which is available in novelty shapes like rockets.

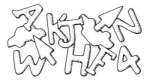

Cook's Tip

For family meals the turkey can be served in the packages but remember to put a dish on the table for the discarded foil! A green salad is a suitable accompaniment.

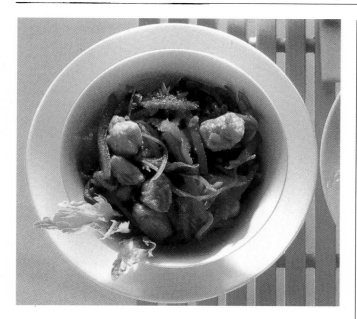

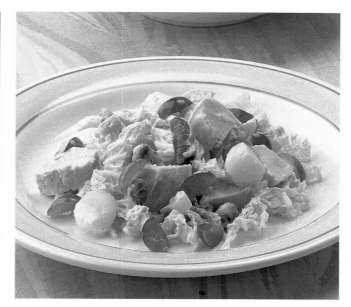

171 | *Diced Turkey with Celery*

Preparation time
25 minutes, plus soaking

Cooking time
3 minutes

Serves 4

Calories
224 per portion

You will need
4 Chinese dried mushrooms
350 g/12 oz boneless turkey breast, skinned and diced
salt
1 egg white
1 tablespoon cornflour
2 tablespoons oil
2 garlic cloves, sliced
2 slices fresh root ginger, finely chopped
2 leeks, diagonally sliced
1 small head celery, diagonally sliced
1 red pepper, seeded and sliced
3 tablespoons light soy sauce
2 tablespoons dry sherry
celery leaves, to garnish

Soak the mushrooms in warm water for 15 minutes. Squeeze dry and discard the stalks, then slice the caps.

Season the diced turkey with salt, dip in the egg white, then coat with cornflour. Heat the oil in a large non-stick frying pan. Add the turkey and stir-fry for 1 minute, until golden brown. Remove with a slotted spoon and drain on absorbent kitchen paper.

Increase the heat, add the garlic, ginger, leeks and celery and stir-fry for 1 minute. Return the turkey to the pan, add the red pepper and stir-fry for 30 seconds. Stir in the soy sauce and sherry and cook for a further 30 seconds. Spoon into a warmed serving dish, garnish with celery leaves and serve immediately.

Cook's Tip

The Chinese learned the art of drying mushrooms many centuries ago, sometimes preserving them in powder form. The mushrooms should be washed in lukewarm water before soaking.

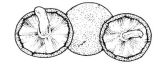

172 | *Turkey Salad*

Preparation time
25 minutes

Serves 4

Calories
330 per portion

You will need
40 g/1½ oz hazelnuts
75 g/3 oz grapes, quartered and pipped
100 g/4 oz drained canned water chestnuts
225 g/8 oz Chinese leaves, finely shredded
450 g/1 lb cooked turkey meat, cut in bite-sized pieces

For the dressing
2 teaspoons grated Parmesan cheese
1 egg
2 teaspoons olive, sunflower or walnut oil
2 teaspoons lemon or orange juice
pinch of mustard powder
1 garlic clove, crushed (optional)
pinch of black pepper
pinch of sea salt
few drops of Worcestershire sauce
150 ml/¼ pint natural low-fat yogurt

Put the hazelnuts in an ungreased heavy-based pan over a low heat for 2-3 minutes, stirring until lightly browned. Combine with all the other salad ingredients in a bowl.

Blend all the dressing ingredients except the yogurt in a liquidizer. Transfer to a jug. Mix the yogurt into the dressing with a wooden spoon and stir the dressing into the salad. Mix well.

Cook's Tip

Turkey is a very lean meat and can become rather dry after cooking. Avoid this happening by covering cooked turkey with stock before storing in the refrigerator if preparing it in advance.

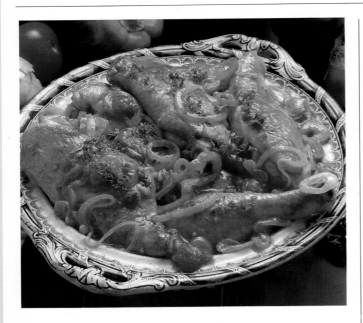

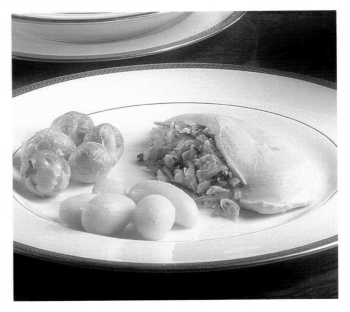

173 | *Turkey Portions Creole*

Preparation time
20 minutes

Cooking time
1½ hours

Serves 6

Calories
209 per portion

You will need
2 tablespoons plain flour
salt and pepper
750 g/1½ lb turkey portions
2 tablespoons oil
2 onions, sliced
1 green pepper, cored and seeded
1 garlic clove, crushed
1 x 400-g/14-oz can peeled
    chopped tomatoes
1 bouquet garni (see Recipe 109)
150 ml/¼ pint chicken stock
chopped parsley, to garnish

Season the flour and use to coat the turkey portions. Heat the oil lightly in a large flameproof casserole and fry the turkey portions until golden on all sides. Add the onion, garlic and green pepper to the turkey, lower the heat and cook gently for 5 minutes. Cook for a minute, then add the tomatoes and juice, bouquet garni and stock. Bring to the boil, stirring, cover tightly and simmer gently for 1¼ hours, or until the turkey portions are tender.

When cooked lift the turkey pieces on to a warmed serving dish and keep hot. Discard the bouquet garni and boil the sauce rapidly, uncovered, until reduced to a coating consistency. Adjust the seasoning to taste and pour over the turkey. Serve sprinkled with parsley.

Cook's Tip

Turkey portions cooked like this make a tasty and economical casserole for family meals. You can always add a little dry white wine to the stock if you want to serve it to guests.

174 | *Turkey Parcels*

Preparation time
35 minutes

Cooking time
35 minutes

Serves 8

Calories
198 per portion

You will need
8 turkey escalopes, about 150 g/
    5 oz each
300 ml/½ pint white wine
300 ml/½ pint turkey or chicken
    stock

For the stuffing
225 g/8 oz courgettes, grated
50 g/2 oz hazelnuts, toasted and
    ground
2 spring onions, trimmed and
    finely chopped
½ tablespoon lime juice
1 teaspoon grated lime rind
1 teaspoon clear honey
1 teaspoon grated fresh ginger
1 teaspoon fresh or dried thyme
coarsely ground black pepper

Prepare the turkey escalopes (see Cook's Tip). Then combine all the stuffing ingredients together in a mixing bowl, adding black pepper to taste. Divide the stuffing between the escalopes, pushing it well into the pockets.

Combine the wine and stock. Pour into one or two large shallow pans and bring to the boil. Reduce to a very gentle simmer and poach the escalopes, stuffing side up, for 20-25 minutes, until cooked through. Remove the escalopes with a slotted spoon and drain on absorbent kitchen paper. Transfer to a warmed serving dish and keep warm.

Boil the poaching liquid fast until reduced to about 150 ml/¼ pint. Spoon a little of the reduced cooking juices over each escalope and serve.

Cook's Tip

Holding a sharp knife horizontally, cut a 5 cm/2 inch slit in each turkey escalope pushing the knife deep into the flesh to make a pocket. Make sure that you do not cut through the flesh.

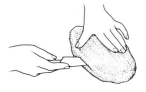

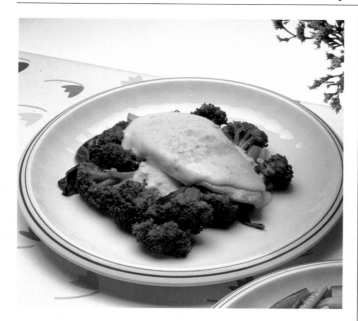

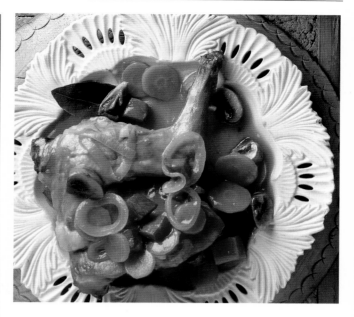

175 | *Turkey with Broccoli*

Preparation time
15 minutes

Cooking time
20-25 minutes

Serves 4

Calories
288 per portion

You will need
4 turkey breasts, about 100 g/4 oz
  each
450 g/1 lb broccoli
salt

For the sauce
25 g/1 oz butter
1 garlic clove, peeled (optional)
2 teaspoons cornflour
300 ml/½ pint skimmed milk
300 ml/½ pint chicken stock
1 bay leaf
25 g/1 oz grated Parmesan cheese

Put the turkey breasts under a preheated hot grill and cook, turning, for about 15 minutes until tender.

Meanwhile, steam the broccoli for about 12 minutes until just tender. Arrange the broccoli on a warmed serving dish and place the turkey breasts on top. Keep hot.

To make the sauce, melt the butter in a saucepan and add the garlic. Cook gently for a few seconds then stir in the cornflour. Cook for 2 minutes, stirring. Remove the garlic. Add enough skimmed milk and chicken stock to make a thin sauce. Add the bay leaf and cook for a few minutes, stirring, until the sauce thickens. Remove the bay leaf. Pour over the turkey breasts and broccoli. Sprinkle with the Parmesan cheese and place under a preheated hot grill until lightly browned.

176 | *Rabbit Casserole*

Preparation time
15 minutes

Cooking time
1 hour 10 minutes

Oven temperature
180°C, 350°F, gas 4

Serves 4

Calories
329 per portion

You will need
750 g/1 ½ lb rabbit joints
150 ml/¼ pint red wine
rind of 1 lemon
2 garlic cloves, crushed
bouquet garni (see Recipe 109)
100 g/4 oz lean cooked ham,
  cubed
225 g/8 oz onions, sliced
225 g/8 oz carrots, thinly sliced
150 g/5 oz button mushrooms,
  halved
1 tablespoon cornflour
¼ teaspoon cayenne
1 tablespoon redcurrant jelly

Put the rabbit, wine, water, lemon rind, garlic, herbs, ham, onion, carrot and salt in a flameproof casserole. Bring to simmering point, cover and cook in the oven for 35 minutes.

Add the mushrooms and cook for 15 minutes, or until the rabbit and vegetables are tender. Using a slotted spoon, transfer meat and vegetables to a warmed serving dish; keep hot.

Mix the cornflour to a smooth paste with a little of the liquid in the casserole. Add to the remaining liquid and cook, stirring over moderate heat, until thickened.

Add the cayenne and redcurrant jelly and cook for 3-4 minutes, until syrupy. Pour over the meat and vegetables.

Cook's Tip

It is very easy to overcook broccoli so watch it carefully. Ideally, it should not have lost its wonderful green colour by the time it is just tender. Try leaving the lid balanced over the top of the steamer to allow some air to reach it.

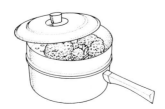

Cook's Tip

Traditionally, dumplings are served with this substantial casserole of the kind that farmers' wives used to make for their menfolk after a day's toil on the land. They would probably have used cider instead of wine.

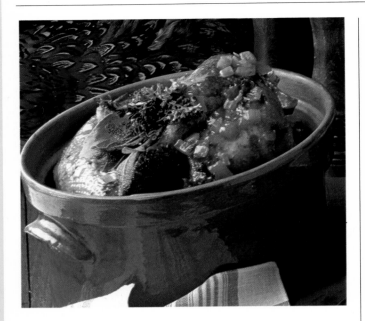

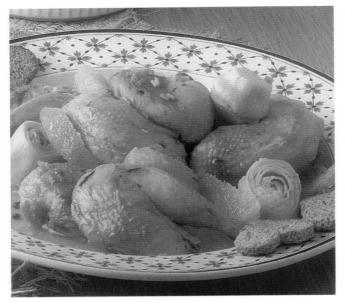

177 | *Faisan en Casserole*

Preparation time
20 minutes

Cooking time
2¾ hours

Oven temperature
160°C, 325°F, gas 3

Serves 6

Calories
491 per portion

You will need
40 g/1 ½ oz butter
1 large pheasant, quartered
2 large onions, chopped
1 garlic clove, crushed
450 ml/¾ pint beef stock
grated rind and juice of 1 orange
150 ml/¼ pint red wine
1 bay leaf
bouquet garni (see Recipe 109)
salt and pepper
2 tablespoons cornflour

Melt the butter in a flameproof casserole, add the pheasant and fry until browned on all sides; remove from the casserole. Add the onions and garlic to the pan and cook gently for 10 minutes. Return the pheasant to the casserole, add the beef stock, orange rind and juice, herbs and salt and pepper to taste. Bring to the boil, then cook in the oven for 2½ hours, or until tender.

Transfer the pheasant to a warmed serving dish; keep hot. Mix the cornflour to a smooth paste with a little of the liquid in the casserole. Add to the remaining liquid and cook, stirring over moderate heat, until thickened. Spoon the sauce over the pheasant to serve.

178 | *Pheasant with Green Peppercorns*

Preparation time
30 minutes, plus
marinating

Cooking time
25-30 minutes

Serves 8

Calories
501 per portion

You will need
2 medium pheasants
175 ml/6 fl oz unsweetened
   orange juice
1 garlic clove, crushed
1 tablespoon chopped chives
salt
2 teaspoons green peppercorns
150 ml/¼ pint dry white wine
4 canned artichoke hearts

For the garnish
heart-shaped croûtons
peeled orange segments

Using a very sharp knife, remove the breasts and drumsticks from each bird. Put the pheasant in a dish with the orange juice, garlic, chives and salt. Cover and chill for 4 hours.

Transfer the pheasant and marinade to a large frying pan. Add the peppercorns and the white wine and simmer for 15-20 minutes. Add the artichoke hearts and simmer for a further 6-8 minutes, until the pheasant is just tender. Remove the pheasant and artichoke hearts and keep warm.

Reduce the cooking juices slightly over a brisk heat; spoon over the pheasant and garnish with the croûtons and orange segments.

Cook's Tip

Unplucked game birds should be hung by the neck in a cool, airy place for between 3 and 10 days after they are shot, before being prepared for either cooking or the freezer.

Cook's Tip

Pheasants with bright, glossy plumage and smooth legs indicate young birds. The cocks should have short spurs. With this information you will be able to impress your poulterer that you are a knowledgeable customer!

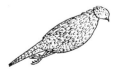

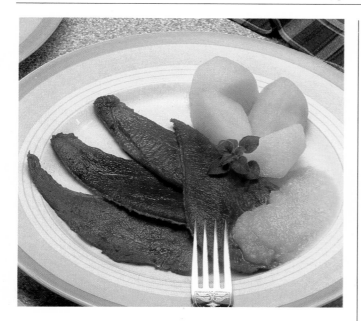

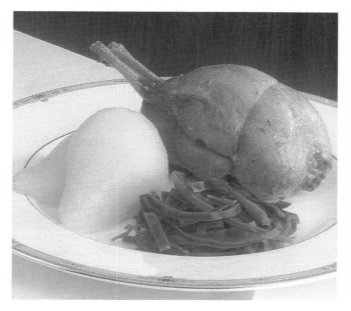

179 | *Wild Duck with Satsuma Sauce*

Preparation time
20 minutes

Cooking time
1 hour 10 minutes

Oven temperature
190°C, 375°F, gas 5

Serves 4

Calories
466 per portion

You will need
5 satsumas
1 small onion, finely chopped
4 tablespoons unsweetened
 orange juice
2 tablespoons dry vermouth
200 ml/7 fl oz chicken stock
salt and pepper
2 wild ducks
4 fresh marjoram sprigs
4 rashers of streaky bacon

Peel the satsumas; separate the segments and remove all the pith. Put the satsuma segments into a pan with the chopped onion, orange juice, vermouth, stock and salt and pepper to taste; simmer gently for 5 minutes. Blend in the liquidizer until smooth.

Sprinkle the ducks inside and out with salt and pepper; put two sprigs of marjoram inside each bird. Stand them in a roasting tin, lay the bacon on the top. Cover the ducks with foil and roast in the oven for 45 minutes. Remove the foil and baste the ducks; return to the oven, uncovered, for about 15 minutes until just tender, but take care not to overcook.

Discard the bacon rashers. Cut off the leg joints from the duck neatly; carve the breasts into thin slices. Heat the satsuma sauce through gently. Serve the wild duck with the sauce spooned over one side.

Cook's Tip

Satsumas have the great advantage of having no pips but they tend to have a lot of pith. If they are not available, you can use other members of the orange family such as mandarins or clementines.

180 | *Partridge with Pears*

Preparation time
30 minutes

Cooking time
45-50 minutes

Oven temperature
200°C, 400°F, gas 6

Serves 10

Calories
283 per portion

You will need
1 sprig fresh rosemary
2 bay leaves
10 cloves
300 ml/½ pint dry white wine
300 ml/½ pint water
10 partridges
salt
1 lemon, quartered
10 firm pears, peeled

Put the herbs and cloves in a saucepan with the wine and water, bring to the boil, cover and remove from the heat while you prepare the birds.

Rub each bird inside and out with salt and a cut lemon. Arrange them in two earthenware oven-to-table dishes, then arrange the pears around the birds.

Bring the wine mixture to the boil again quickly and pour over the birds and pears. Put in the oven. Cook for 45-50 minutes if both dishes fit on the centre shelf. If not, put the dishes on different shelves for 20 minutes, then swap them for the next 20 minutes. Change them over again for a further 15 minutes, then take the top dish out and keep it warm while you give the other dish a final 20 minutes in the centre of the oven. During cooking, check that the liquids do not dry up, topping up with more water if necessary. Serve one pear and a little of the cooking juice with each partridge.

Cook's Tip

When choosing a partridge, look for yellow legs and sharp-pointed long wing feathers. Once the feathers are rounded, the bird is old and past its prime. You should therefore preferably choose birds before they are plucked.

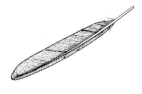

Vegetables and Salads

The marvellous selection of vegetables available today means it is possible to create colourful, exciting salads and cooked vegetable dishes all the year round. Try cooking some of the more unusual vegetable recipes in this chapter such as Celeriac Sticks in Mustard Sauce. Using herbs and spices in sauces and dressings enhances the subtle flavours of vegetables, while pulses provide valuable protein and fibre.

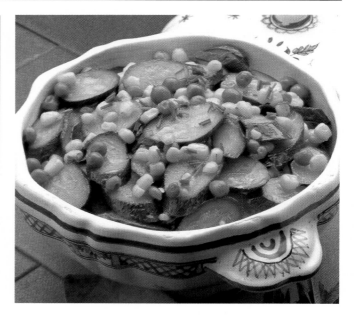

181 | Orange Winter Salad

Preparation time
20 minutes

Serves 4

Calories
278 per portion

You will need
4 large oranges
1 x 400-g/14-oz can red kidney
    beans, drained
275 g/10 oz beansprouts
4 celery sticks, trimmed, scrubbed
    and thinly sliced
watercress sprigs, to garnish

For the light French dressing
3 tablespoons olive oil
2 tablespoons lemon juice
salt
¼ teaspoon sugar
freshly ground black pepper
¼ teaspoon made English
    mustard

Using a serrated knife, cut the top and bottom from the oranges, then remove all the skin and pith, leaving a ball of fruit. Cut into segments by cutting down on either side of each membrane, and put in a bowl with any juice that runs out while cutting. Add the beans, beansprouts and celery and toss lightly together.

To make the dressing, put all the ingredients into a screw-topped jar and shake vigorously until blended.

Just before serving the salad spoon the dressing over and garnish with watercress.

182 | Minted Courgettes with Peas and Corn

Preparation time
5 minutes

Cooking time
6-7 minutes

Serves 2

Calories
53 per portion

You will need
175 g/6 oz courgettes, thinly sliced
    salt
50 g/2 oz frozen peas
50 g/2 oz frozen sweetcorn
2 mint sprigs
2 teaspoons chopped chives

Put the courgettes in a pan of boiling lightly salted water. Add the peas, sweetcorn and mint. Cover and simmer for 5-6 minutes until the vegetables are just tender. Drain, remove the mint and return the vegetables to the pan. Add the chives and toss to combine evenly.

Transfer to a warmed serving dish. Serve hot.

Cook's Tip

This crisp colourful salad is both delicious and nutritious. The watercress must be rinsed thoroughly in cold water and any discoloured leaves discarded. Break off the coarser stems as these are rather peppery.

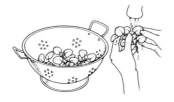

Cook's Tip

Double the quantities of vegetables and reserve half to include in a salad. If you are serving the courgettes with a low-calorie main course, try tossing the drained vegetables with a little butter.

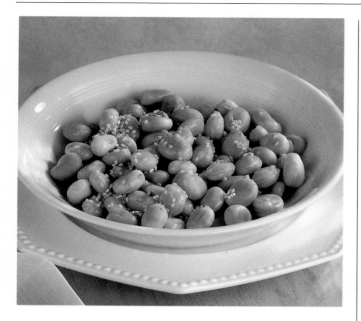

183 | Broad Beans with Sesame

Preparation time
5-15 minutes

Cooking time
8-15 minutes

Serves 4

Calories
191 per portion

You will need
450 g/1 lb broad beans, prepared
weight, fresh or frozen
2 tablespoons sesame seeds
15 g/½ oz butter
1 tablespoon lemon juice
freshly ground black pepper

Cook the beans in boiling lightly salted water until tender, 8-15 minutes depending on whether fresh or frozen.

Meanwhile toast the sesame seeds under a moderate grill to brown them evenly.

Drain the beans, and put the butter in the pan. Melt it quickly and when just beginning to brown add the lemon juice and pepper. Tip the beans back into the pan and toss well in the butter.

Serve sprinkled with the sesame seeds.

184 | Lemon Cabbage with Poppy Seeds

Preparation time
15 minutes

Cooking time
12 minutes

Serves 4

Calories
53 per portion

You will need
150 ml/¼ pint water
salt
350 g/12 oz green cabbage,
shredded
350 g/12 oz hard white cabbage,
shredded
15 g/½ oz butter, cut into small
pieces
grated rind of 1 lemon
1 ½ teaspoons poppy seeds
freshly ground black pepper
2 tablespoons smetana, to serve
(optional)

Put the water into a large saucepan, add a little salt and bring to the boil. Add both green and white cabbage, cover and simmer steadily for 7-10 minutes. The cabbage should be crisply tender and most of the water absorbed.

Take the lid off the pan and boil quickly to reduce any remaining liquid. Add the pieces of butter, lemon rind, poppy seeds and lots of black pepper. Stir briefly until the butter is melted and the cabbage evenly coated.

Spoon the hot cabbage into a warm dish and serve with smetana spooned over the top, if liked.

Cook's Tip

If you are using fresh broad beans, you may find some of the pods are a little discoloured. The actual beans inside can be perfect so do not discard without splitting the pod open to check.

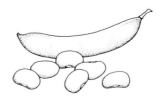

Cook's Tip

The colour contrast of the green and white cabbage gives this simple vegetable dish an attractive appearance. It can be served with a wide variety of meat or poultry dishes.

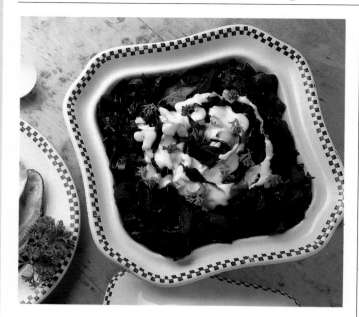

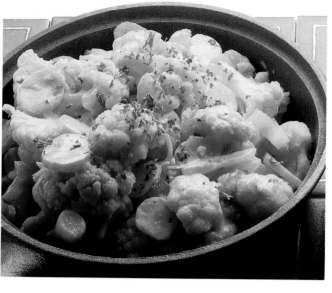

185 | *Spicy Red Cabbage*

Preparation time
10 minutes

Cooking time
8-12 minutes

Serves 4

Calories
40 per portion

You will need
1 medium red cabbage, shredded
1 tablespoon vinegar
2 teaspoons caraway seeds
¼ teaspoon ground allspice
1 tablespoon smetana
parsley sprig, to garnish

Rinse the cabbage under cold running water. Pour boiling water into a large saucepan to a depth of 1 cm/½ inch and add the cabbage, vinegar, caraway seeds and allspice.

Cover tightly and cook over a moderate heat for 8-12 minutes, stirring occasionally until the cabbage is tender.

Drain the cabbage thoroughly and transfer to a heated serving dish. Serve hot with the smetana spooned over the top, garnished with parsley.

186 | *Spiced Cauliflower*

Preparation time
15 minutes

Cooking time
15 minutes

Serves 4

Calories
82 per portion

You will need
1 tablespoon oil
1 teaspoon ground ginger
2 teaspoons ground coriander
1 teaspoon ground turmeric
1 onion, sliced
1 cauliflower, broken into florets
2 carrots, thinly sliced
2 celery sticks, sliced
120 ml/4 fl oz stock
salt and pepper
150 ml/¼ pint natural low-fat
  yogurt
1 tablespoon chopped coriander or
  parsley

Heat the oil in a pan, add the spices and fry gently for 1 minute. Add the onion and cook gently for a further 3 minutes, stirring occasionally. Add the remaining vegetables, the stock, and salt and pepper to taste.

Cover and simmer for about 10 minutes until the vegetables are just tender. Stir in the yogurt, sprinkle with the coriander or parsley and serve immediately.

Cook's Tip

Discard any limp outer leaves before shredding the red cabbage. Smetana is a low-fat substitute for cream with a slightly sour taste that also combines well with soft fruit. It is available in most supermarkets.

Cook's Tip

Frying the spices gently brings out their flavour and aroma. It is important not to overcook the vegetables which should still be quite crunchy. Use either a chicken or vegetable stock.

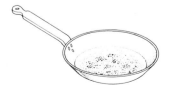

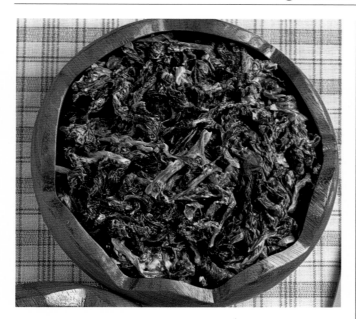

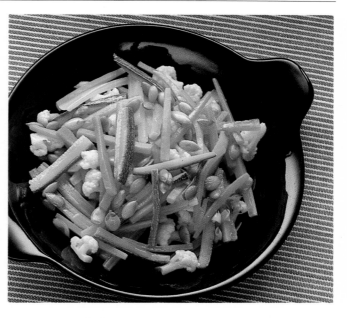

187 | *Spinach with Yogurt*

Preparation time
5-10 minutes

Cooking time
5-10 minutes

Serves 4

Calories
100 per portion

You will need
1 kg/2¼ lb fresh spinach
150 ml/¼ pint natural low-fat
   yogurt
1-2 garlic cloves, crushed
salt and pepper

Rinse the spinach thoroughly in cold water and cook in a covered pan, without additional water, until tender. Shake the pan occasionally. Drain and leave to cool.

   Mix together the yogurt and garlic and stir into the spinach. Add salt and pepper to taste. Transfer to a warmed serving dish.

188 | *Mixed Vegetable Stir-fry*

Preparation time
20 minutes

Cooking time
10 minutes

Serves 4

Calories
124 per portion

You will need
1 cauliflower, about 350 g/12 oz
2 carrots, about 100 g/4 oz
2 courgettes, about 175 g/6 oz
2 celery sticks
1 tablespoon vegetable oil
15 g/½ oz butter
2 tablespoons pumpkin seeds
salt and pepper

Break the cauliflower into very small florets. Cut the carrots into thin strips about 4 cm x 3 mm/1½ x ⅛ inch. Cut the courgettes into chunks, then into strips like the carrots. Trim the celery and cut into 4 cm/1½ inch lengths, then into strips in the same way.

   Heat the oil and butter together in a large non-stick frying pan or wok. Add the pumpkin seeds and fry for about 1 minute, taking care as they will jump about in the heat.

   Add all the vegetables at once, sprinkle with salt and pepper and cook over a steady heat, shaking the pan and turning the vegetables lightly for about 8-10 minutes until crisply tender. Serve immediately.

Cook's Tip

Frozen leaf spinach may be used if fresh spinach is not available. You will need 500 g/ 1¼ lb. Cook it according to the instructions on the packet. Reserve the liquid to give flavour to a soup made from leftover vegetables.

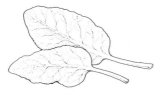

Cook's Tip

This is one of the best way to cook vegetables. The colours stay bright and the quick cooking without water retains all the goodness. You can use other combinations of vegetables but always cut them in tiny pieces to ensure **that they cook quickly and remain crisp.**

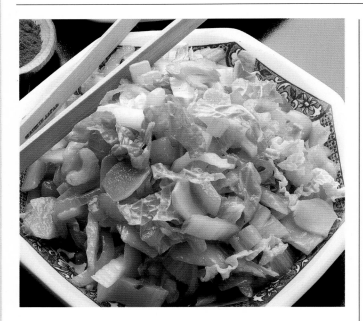

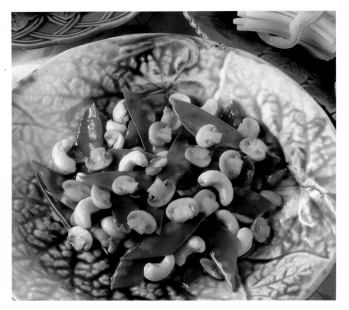

189 | *Stir-fried Chinese Leaves*

Preparation time
15 minutes

Cooking time
8 minutes

Serves 4

Calories
82 per portion

You will need
8-10 stems Chinese leaves
100 g/4 oz bamboo shoots, sliced
1 onion, sliced
1 celery stick, sliced
2 tablespoons oil
lemon juice
salt and pepper

Cut the Chinese leaves diagonally into 3 mm/⅛ inch strips.

Heat the oil in a non-stick frying pan or wok. Add the vegetables and fry gently for about 8 minutes, stirring frequently. Add a little lemon juice and seasoning to taste.

190 | *Stir-fried Mushrooms*

Preparation time
15 minutes

Cooking time
7-8 minutes

Serves 4

Calories
140 per portion

You will need
225 g/8 oz mangetout, topped,
    tailed and cut diagonally into
    4 cm/1 ½ inch slices
salt
2 tablespoons vegetable oil
1 garlic clove, crushed
225 g/8 oz button mushrooms,
    sliced
25 g/1 oz cashew nuts

For the sauce
2 tablespoons soy sauce
2 tablespoons dry sherry
5 tablespoons chicken stock
1 teaspoon clear honey
pinch of cayenne

Cook the mangetout slices in boiling lightly salted water for 2 minutes. Drain them, then plunge them immediately into ice cold water to prevent further cooking and to preserve their colour. Drain and dry with absorbent kitchen paper.

Mix all the sauce ingredients in a bowl.

Heat the oil in a heavy-based non-stick frying pan or wok and stir-fry the garlic with a pinch of salt over a high heat for 1 minute. Add the mangetout slices and the mushrooms and stir-fry them for 2 minutes.

Pour on the sauce, bring to the boil and cook for 2-3 minutes until the sauce has almost evaporated and the vegetables are just tender and glistening. Add the cashews and just heat through. Serve at once.

Cook's Tip

If you only need a few drops of lemon juice, pierce the end of the fruit with a cocktail stick and squeeze gently. Then wrap the lemon tightly in cling film and keep in the refrigerator until needed.

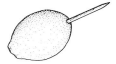

Cook's Tip

As their French name implies, the pods of mangetout peas are edible. They tend to be rather expensive so try growing some if you are lucky enough to have a garden.

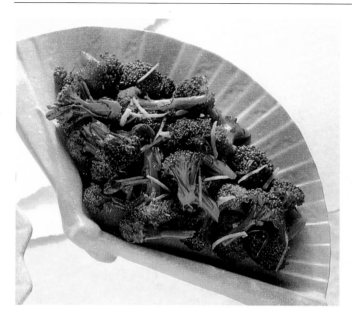

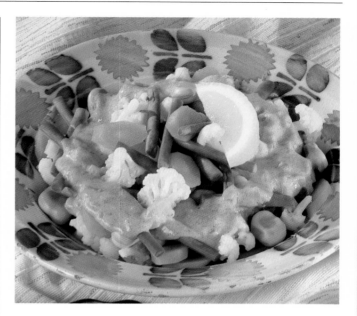

191 | *Stir-fried Ginger Broccoli*

Preparation time
10 minutes

Cooking time
3-4 minutes

Serves 4

Calories
107 per portion

You will need
500 g/1 ¼ lb broccoli
salt
2 tablespoons oil
1 garlic clove, thinly sliced
(optional)
1 x 2.5 cm/1 inch piece fresh root
ginger, finely shredded
½-1 teaspoon sesame oil

Separate the broccoli heads into small florets, and peel and diagonally slice the stems. Blanch in boiling lightly salted water for 30 seconds, drain well and cool rapidly under cold running water; drain thoroughly.

Heat the oil in a large non-stick frying pan or wok, add the garlic and ginger and stir-fry for 2-3 seconds. Add the blanched broccoli and cook for 2 minutes. Sprinkle over the sesame oil and stir fry for a further 30 seconds.

Spoon into a warmed serving dish and serve immediately.

192 | *Vegetables in Curry Sauce*

Preparation time
20 minutes

Cooking time
25 minutes

Serves 4

Calories
166 per portion

You will need
1 small cauliflower, cut into florets
225 g/8 oz carrots, thinly sliced
225 g/8 oz shelled broad beans
225 g/8 oz young French beans,
topped, tailed and halved
450 m/¾ pint vegetable stock

For the sauce
1 tablespoon oil
1 small onion, chopped
2 teaspoons curry paste
1 tablespoon wholemeal flour
150 ml/¼ pint natural low-fat
yogurt
1 teaspoon lemon juice
salt and pepper

Cook the vegetables in a covered steamer over the stock for 12 minutes, or simmer them in the stock for 9-10 minutes until they are just tender. Drain the vegetables and reserve the stock.

To make the sauce, heat the oil in a non-stick saucepan and fry the onion over a moderate heat for 3 minutes, stirring occasionally. Stir in the curry powder and curry paste and cook for 1 minute. Stir in the flour and cook for 2 minutes. Measure 275 ml/9 fl oz of the reserved stock and gradually pour it on to the curry mixture, stirring constantly. Gradually stir in the yogurt, then add the lemon juice and season with salt and pepper. Bring the sauce to the boil slowly and simmer for 2-3 minutes.

Put the vegetables in a dish and stir in the sauce.

Cook's Tip

The character of garlic changes according to the way in which it is cooked. It becomes quite mild and almost sweet in a slow-cooked casserole but if it is fried to a nutty brown, it is much more pungent.

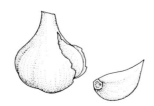

Cook's Tip

Since the strict Hindu does not eat meat, much authentic Indian cooking is vegetarian. If you serve some plain boiled rice with these curried vegetables, they will form a nutritious main course.

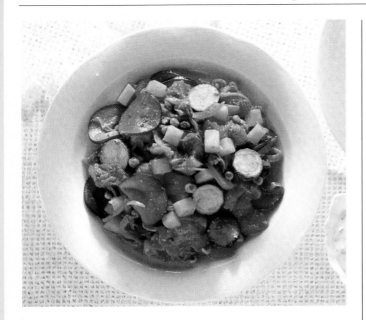

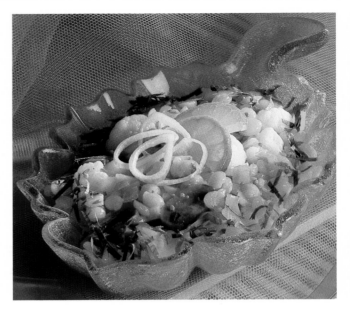

193 | Indian Vegetable Medley

Preparation time
20 minutes

Cooking time
35 minutes

Serves 4

Calories
142 per portion

You will need
3 tablespoons oil
1 teaspoon fennel seeds
2 onions, sliced
1 teaspoon ground coriander
1 teaspoon cumin seeds
1 teaspoon chilli powder
2 teaspoons finely chopped fresh
  root ginger
2 garlic cloves, crushed
1 small aubergine, thinly sliced
1 potato, cubed
1 green pepper, seeded and sliced
2 courgettes, sliced
1 x 400-g/14-oz can tomatoes
2 green chillies, chopped,
  including seeds
salt
50 g/2 oz frozen peas

Heat the oil in a large non-stick frying pan or wok, stir in the fennel seeds and cook for 1 minute, stirring constantly. Add the onion and cook for 5 minutes, until pale brown. Lower the heat, add all the spices and cook, stirring, for 1 minute. Add the ginger, garlic, aubergine and potato, mix well and cook for 15 minutes. Add the green pepper, courgettes, tomatoes with their juice, chillies and salt. Bring to the boil slowly and then simmer for 10 minutes, stirring occasionally.

Stir in the peas and cook for 3 minutes, until the vegetables are tender and the liquid absorbed. Transfer to a warmed serving dish and serve immediately.

Cook's Tip

This vegetable medley will appeal to people who enjoy a fiery taste. Accompany with a little natural low-fat yogurt for those who prefer milder flavours. Don't forget to put a large jug of iced water on the table.

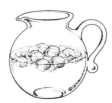

194 | Ginger Dal

Preparation time
20 minutes

Cooking time
1 hour

Serves 4

Calories
122 per portion

You will need
225 g/8 oz yellow split peas (see
  Cook's Tip)
600 ml/1 pint chicken or vegetable
  stock
175 g/6 oz cauliflower florets
1 tablespoon vegetable oil
½ teaspoon mustard seeds
½ teaspoon fennel seeds
1 teaspoon chopped fresh root
  ginger
1 small onion, chopped
100 g/4 oz button mushrooms,
  thinly sliced
salt and pepper

For the garnish
2 tablespoons chopped fresh
  coriander or parsley
lime slices
1 small onion, sliced into rings

Put the split peas and stock into a saucepan, bring to the boil, cover and simmer for about 45 minutes or until the split peas are tender. Meanwhile, steam the cauliflower florets for 10 minutes until they are beginning to soften.

Heat the oil in a small saucepan and fry the mustard, fennel seeds and ginger over a moderate heat for 1 minute, stirring. Add the onion and fry for 3-4 minutes, stirring. Add the onion mixture, the cauliflower and mushrooms to the pulses and season. Simmer for 5 minutes.

Turn the dal into a warmed dish. Sprinkle on the herb and arrange the lime slices and onion rings on top.

Cook's Tip

Rinse the split peas thoroughly in cold water to remove any impurities and drain in a sieve before cooking. Unlike other pulses, neither lentils nor split peas need to be soaked overnight.

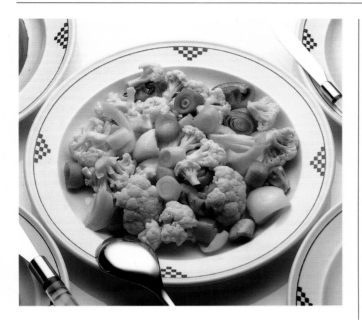

195 | Oriental Vegetables

Preparation time
15 minutes

Cooking time
20 minutes

Serves 4

Calories
57 per portion

You will need
450 g/1 lb mixed vegetables (see
    Cook's Tip)
120 ml/4 fl oz dry white wine
120 ml/4 fl oz wine vinegar
1 teaspoon coriander
1 teaspoon ground mace
1 teaspoon dried rosemary
salt

Put all the prepared vegetables in a suacepan with the white wine, vinegar, spices, rosemary and salt. Add enough water to cover, bring to the boil and simmer gently for 15-20 minutes. The vegetables should be slightly crisp. Serve hot or cold.

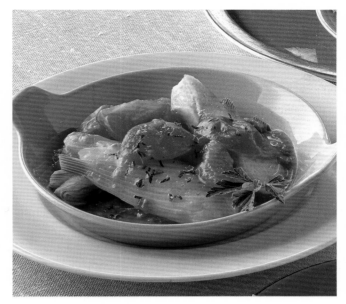

196 | Fennel in Wine Sauce

Preparation time
10 minutes

Cooking time
20-25 minutes

Serves 4

Calories
138 per portion

You will need
2-3 large heads fennel
2 teaspoons olive oil
2 garlic cloves, halved
300 ml/½ pint meat or vegetable
    stock
300 ml/½ pint dry white wine
3 tomatoes, cut into wedges
1 bay leaf
3 peppercorns
salt
sugar
pinch of curry powder
2 tablespoons coarsely chopped
    parsley
1 teaspoon cornflour

Remove the stalks from the fennel and cut the heads into quarters.

Heat the oil in a non-stick pan. Add the garlic and fry until golden brown. Remove and discard the garlic. Add the stock and wine to the pan, stirring well. Add the fennel, tomatoes, bay leaf and peppercorns. Season with salt and sugar to taste. Simmer over a low heat for 15-20 minutes. Add the curry powder and parsley, blending well. Discard the bay leaf.

Dissolve the cornflour in 2 teaspoons water. Add to the fennel mixture, stirring constantly. Cook, stirring, for 1-2 minutes. Transfer to a warmed serving dish and serve immediately.

Cook's Tip

Try a mixture of cauliflower florets, onions cut into eighths, sliced leeks and sliced fennel. Remember to combine vegetables which take a similar cooking time or add the one which needs least time a little later.

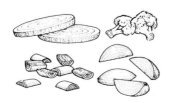

Cook's Tip

Fennel with its slight taste of aniseed can also be cooked in a number of other ways which are suitable for celery or celeriac, such as braising or steaming whole. It is available throughout the winter.

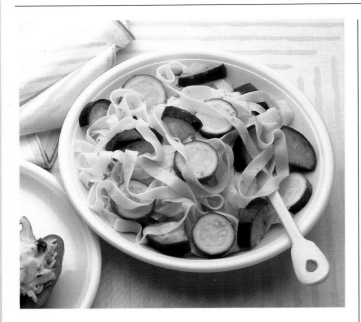

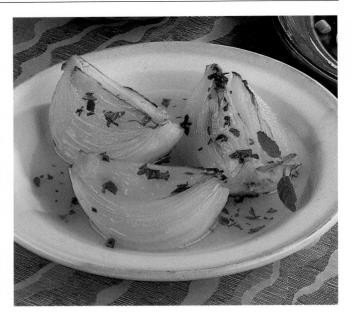

197 | Persian Noodles

Preparation time
10 minutes, plus
draining

Cooking time
16-20 minutes

Serves 4

Calories
120 per portion

You will need
1 large aubergine, thickly sliced
salt and pepper
600 ml/1 pint chicken stock
100 g/4 oz noodles
4 courgettes, sliced
1 teaspoon ground mace

Place the aubergine slices in a colander set over a plate, sprinkle with the salt and set aside to drain for 30 minutes.

Rinse the augergine in cold water, drain and pat dry with absorbent kitchen paper, then chop into bite-sized pieces.

Place the stock in a large saucepan and bring to the boil. Add the noodles and cook for 5 minutes, then add the aubergine, courgettes, mace and pepper to taste.

Reduce the heat and cook for a further 10-15 minutes, or until the noodles and vegetables are tender. Adjust the seasoning to taste, drain and pile into a heated serving dish and serve.

198 | Braised Onions in Cider and Sage

Preparation time
10 minutes

Cooking time
1¼ hours

Oven temperature
180°C, 350°F, gas 4

Serves 4

Calories
82 per portion

You will need
2 large Spanish onions, about
    450 g/1 lb total weight
1 tablespoon vegetable oil
300 ml/½ pint dry cider
salt and pepper
2 teaspoons chopped fresh sage
    or ½ teaspoon dried sage
1 teaspoon cornflour
1 tablespoon water

Remove the papery skins from the onions and cut each into quarters. Trim the bases very lightly so that the quarters stay intact during cooking. Heat the oil in a non-stick frying pan and quickly fry the onion quarters on all sides until golden brown. Put the onions in a small shallow casserole, cut side up. Pour the cider into the pan with the salt, pepper and sage. Bring to the boil, then pour over the onions. Cover the casserole and cook in the oven for 40 minutes.

Remove from the oven, blend the cornflour with the water and stir into the liquor surrounding the onions. Cover again and replace in the oven for a further 20 minutes, by which time the onions will be tender and the sauce slightly thickened. Serve hot.

Cook's Tip

Mace comes from the nutmeg: it is, in fact, the net-like covering on the nutmeg. It is used either whole or ground to a fine powder.

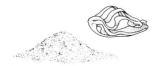

Cook's Tip

Vegetables cooked in their own sauce like these braised onions are ideal for serving with any lean meat or poultry. It is a time-saving method too as you will not need to make any gravy.

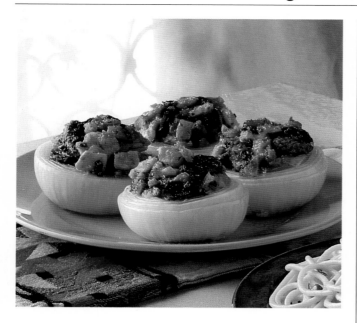

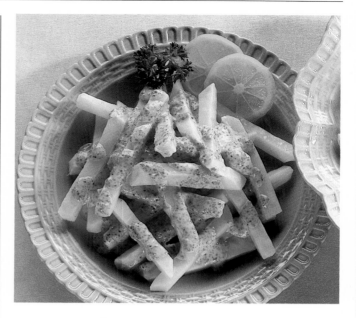

199 | *Stuffed Spanish Onions*

Preparation time
20 minutes

Cooking time
40 minutes

Oven temperature
220°C, 425°F, gas 7

Serves 4

Calories
79 per portion

You will need
2 large Spanish onions, halved
salt and pepper
15 g/½ oz butter
50 g/2 oz lean smoked bacon,
    derinded and chopped
3 tomatoes, peeled and chopped
150 g/5 oz button mushrooms,
    sliced
1 tablespoon chopped parsley
1 tablespoon grated Parmesan
    cheese
1-2 teaspoons dried oregano

Scoop a hollow in the centre of each onion half with a teaspoon, reserving the scooped out onion. Place the halves in a saucepan and cover with water. Add a little salt, bring to the boil and cook for about 15 minutes, until almost tender. Drain well.

Meanwhile, chop the reserved onion. Melt the butter in a non-stick frying pan and cook the bacon and onion for 4-5 minutes. Add the tomatoes and mushrooms and cook for a further 2-3 minutes. Remove the pan from the heat, stir in the parsley and cheese and season to taste with salt, pepper and oregano.

Fill the onion halves with this mixture and put in an ovenproof dish. Cover the base of the dish with water to a depth of 1 cm/½ inch. Cook in the oven for 12-15 minutes.

Cook's Tip

Check the onions for tenderness after they have been boiled for about 15 minutes. The time will, of course, depend on how much onion you have scooped out from the centres.

200 | *Celeriac Sticks with Mustard*

Preparation time
15 minutes

Cooking time
25 minutes

Serves 6

Calories
49 per portion

You will need
750 g/1½ lb celeriac
salt
1 tablespoon lemon juice

For the dressing
150 ml/¼ pint natural low-fat
    yogurt
freshly ground black pepper
1 tablespoon wholegrain mustard

For the garnish
lemon slices
coriander leaves or parsley sprigs

Peel the celeriac and cut first into thick slices, then into chips about 7.5 x 1 cm/3 x ½ inch. Put the chips into a pan with a pinch of salt and the lemon juice and cover with water. Bring to the boil, cover the pan and simmer for 15-20 minutes until the celeriac is tender but still firm. Drain and keep warm in a serving dish.

Pour the yogurt into the rinsed-out pan and stir in the salt, pepper and mustard. Heat very gently until hot, taking care that it does not boil. Pour the cream and mustard dressing over the celeriac and garnish with lemon slices and the coriander leaves or parsley. Serve immediately.

Cook's Tip

Celeriac looks rather like a knobbly swede. It tastes rather like celery and it has a texture rather like a turnip. It can also be served cold with French dressing as a starter.

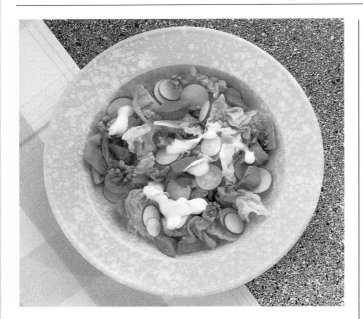

201 | Chicken Liver and Walnut Salad

Preparation time
15 minutes

Cooking time
10 minutes

Serves 4

Calories
254 per portion

You will need
5 teaspoons walnut or olive oil
450 g/1 lb chicken livers
25 g/1 oz walnut pieces
1 garlic clove, crushed (optional)
2 teaspoons wine vinegar
3 tablespoons natural low-fat
  yogurt
salt and pepper
½ lettuce, washed and torn into
  pieces
50 g/2 oz radishes, trimmed and
  very thinly sliced
4 spring onions, trimmed and
  finely chopped

Brush a thick saucepan with 1 teaspoon of the oil and heat gently. With kitchen scissors snip the chicken livers into quarters, directly into the pan, cutting off and discarding any green parts. Stir over a medium heat for 4 minutes. Add the walnut pieces, turn the heat down as low as possible, cover tightly and simmer for a further 5 minutes. The livers should be just cooked and still slightly pink inside.

Meanwhile, blend the remaining oil with the garlic (if using), vinegar, yogurt, salt and pepper in a jug. Place the lettuce, radishes and spring onions in a bowl and toss.

Divide the vegetable mixture among four shallow bowls or dinner plates. Spoon the liver quarters with the walnuts and pan juices over the vegetables and serve, accompanied by the dressing.

Cook's Tip

Although walnut oil is expensive, it is well worth using it rather than olive oil to give the authentic flavour to this unusual warm salad. The juices from the chicken liver combine deliciously with the crunchy vegetables.

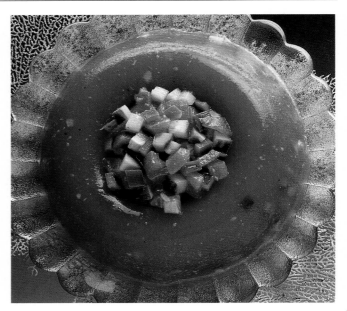

202 | Gazpacho Ring

Preparation time
20 minutes, plus chilling

Cooking time
8 minutes

Serves 6

Calories
43 per portion

You will need
1 x 400-g/14-oz can tomatoes
2 garlic cloves, chopped
150 ml/¼ pint water
bouquet garni (see Recipe 109)
salt and pepper
1 tablespoon powdered gelatine
4 tablespoons water
2 tablespoons light French
  dressing (see Recipe 181)

For the salad
4 tomatoes, peeled, seeded and
  diced
¼ cucumber, diced
½ green pepper, seeded and
  diced
½ onion, finely chopped

Put the tomatoes, with their juice, in a saucepan with the garlic, water and bouquet garni. Add salt and pepper to taste. Bring slowly to the boil, then simmer for 5 minutes. Discard the bouquet garni.

Dissolve the gelatine with the water in a small bowl over a pan of gently simmering water.

Put the tomato mixture in a blender or food processor. Add the gelatine and blend on maximum speed for 30 seconds. Leave to cool.

Add half the salad ingredients and stir well. Turn into a 750 ml/1 ¼ pint non-stick ring mould and chill for about 3 hours, or until set. Mix the remaining salad ingredients with the French dressing. Turn out the tomato ring on to a serving plate and place the salad in the centre.

Cook's Tip

Instead of just using the remaining salad ingredients in the centre of the gazpacho ring, add some lean chopped chicken or white fish to make a main course dish and accompany with a crisp green salad.

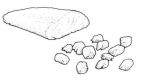

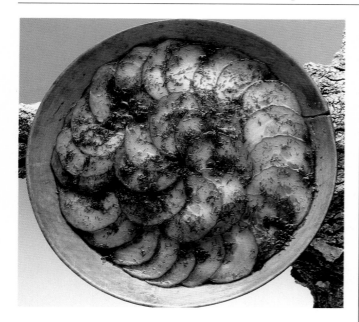

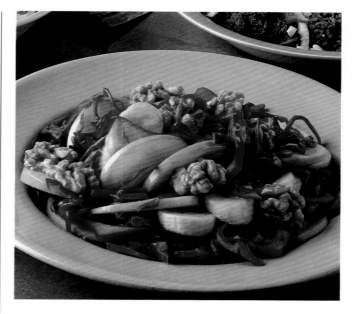

203 | *Swedish Cucumber Salad*

Preparation time
10 minutes, plus
draining

Serves 6

Calories
28 per portion

You will need
1 cucumber
salt

For the dressing
1 tablespoon clear honey
1 tablespoon water
2 tablespoons chopped dill or
  fennel
4 tablespoons white wine vinegar

Slice the cucumber very thinly and place in a colander. Sprinkle liberally with salt and leave to drain for 30 minutes.

Meanwhile, mix the dressing ingredients together in a screw-topped jar. Shake well and leave for 30 minutes.

Dry the cucumber thoroughly on absorbent kitchen paper. Arrange the cucumber slices overlapping in a shallow dish and pour over the dressing.

204 | *Roman Red Cabbage Salad*

Preparation time
15 minutes, plus
standing

Cooking time
5 minutes

Serves 4

Calories
138 per portion

You will need
3 teaspoons lemon juice
2 bananas, peeled and sliced
1 apple, cored and sliced
1 medium red cabbage, shredded
15 g/½ oz walnut halves
2 tablespoons red wine vinegar
2 teaspoons honey
salt and pepper

Sprinkle the lemon juice over the banana and apple slices to prevent discolouration. Mix the cabbage with the banana, apple and walnuts in a serving bowl.

To make the dressing, heat the vinegar in a small pan until warm and add the honey, stirring well to dissolve. Season with salt and pepper to taste. Leave until cool.

Pour the dressing over the red cabbage mixture, and toss well. Leave the salad to stand for a few minutes before serving to allow the flavours to develop.

Cook's Tip

Cucumber salad is the perfect choice to serve with either hot or cold fish. The addition of either dill or fennel also makes the dressing particularly suitable as an accompaniment to a fish dish.

Cook's Tip

This salad is particularly good served with pheasant. Red cabbage is easily obtainable during the winter months and is far less expensive than green salad leaves. The honey in the dressing brings out the flavour.

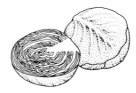

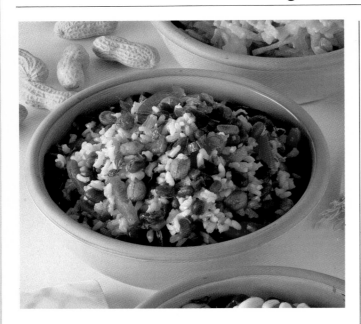

205 | Mixed Bean and Corn Salad

Preparation time
15 minutes, plus soaking and standing

Cooking time
45 minutes

Serves 4

Calories
221 per portion

You will need
75 g/3 oz red kidney beans, soaked overnight
75 g/3 oz haricot beans, soaked overnight
75 g/3 oz fresh or frozen green beans
1 x 200-g/7-oz can sweetcorn, drained
1 tablespoon chopped mixed herbs or 2 teaspoons dried herbs
4 tablespoons light French dressing (see Recipe 181)

Drain the kidney and haricot beans, rinse and place in separate pans. Cover the cold water and bring to the boil. Cook rapidly for 10 minutes, then reduce the heat and cook for 30-35 minutes, or until the beans are tender. Drain and place in a serving bowl.

Cook the green and broad beans in boiling water until tender, then drain and add to the serving bowl. Stir in the sweetcorn and herbs. Pour the French dressing over the salad, then mix well. If possible, add the dressing while the beans are still warm and leave at room temperature for 1-2 hours before serving.

Cook's Tip

You can save time by using drained canned kidney and haricot beans but remember to rinse these thoroughly under cold running water. Check the labels on the cans to see what additives have been included.

206 | Savoy Salad

Preparation time
15 minutes

Cooking time
2 minutes

Serves 4

Calories
114 per portion

You will need
1 teaspoon caraway seeds
2 tablespoons olive or sunflower oil
2 teaspoons lemon juice
1 teaspoon red wine vinegar
1 teaspoon mild mustard
pinch of pepper
pinch of salt
100 g/4 oz cottage or smooth low-fat soft cheese
2 tablespoons water
225 g/8 oz Savoy cabbage, very finely shredded
100 g/4 oz red or green pepper, seeded and finely diced

Put the caraway seeds in an ungreased heavy-based frying pan and stir over a low heat for 1-2 minutes. Crush in an electric coffee mill or with a mortar and pestle.

Transfer to a blender and add the oil, lemon juice, vinegar, mustard, pepper, salt, cheese and water. Blend the dressing until smooth.

Place the prepared cabbage and pepper in a serving bowl and stir well. Spoon the dressing over and serve.

Cook's Tip

If you are using an electric coffee mill to crush the caraway seeds, first grind a slice of bread. This will remove any fragments of coffee beans that may be trapped under the blade.

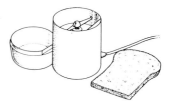

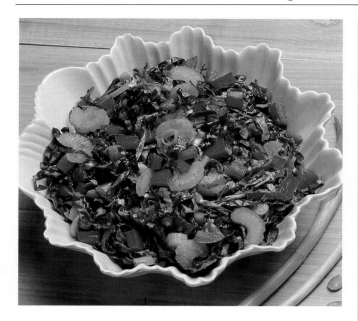

207 | *Spring Cabbage and Pepper Salad*

Preparation time
15 minutes, plus marinating

Serves 6

Calories
57 per portion

You will need
250 g/9 oz spring cabbage, shredded
4 tablespoons light French dressing (see Recipe 181)
1 teaspoon light soy sauce
3 celery sticks, sliced
4 spring onions, chopped
1 red pepper, seeded and diced

Combine the dressing with the soy sauce. Put the spring cabbage in a bowl with the dressing, toss thoroughly and leave to marinate for 1 hour.

Add the remaining ingredients and toss thoroughly. Transfer to a salad bowl to serve.

Cook's Tip

Spring cabbage is an unusual ingredient for a salad. Pick over the leaves carefully, discarding any that are blemished. Make this salad the same day as you obtain the spring cabbage as the leaves soon become limp.

208 | *Charlotte d'Aubergines*

Preparation time
20 minutes, plus standing

Cooking time
1½ hours

Oven temperature
180°C, 350°F, gas 4

Serves 6

Calories
122 per portion

You will need
1 kg/2¼ lb aubergines, sliced
salt
15 g/½ oz butter
1 large onion, sliced
2 garlic cloves, crushed
500 g/1¼ lb tomatoes, peeled and chopped
2 tablespoons oil
300 ml/½ pint natural low-fat yogurt
150 ml/¼ pint chicken stock

Sprinkle the aubergine slices with salt and leave to stand for 30 minutes. Rinse under cold water and dry thoroughly with absorbent kitchen paper.

Melt the butter in a non-stick frying pan, add the onion and garlic and fry until lightly browned. Stir in the tomatoes and cook for 20-25 minutes, until thickened.

Heat the oil in another non-stick pan and fry the aubergine slices until browned on both sides. Drain thoroughly on absorbent kitchen paper.

Line the base and sides of a 1.5 litre/2 ½ pint charlotte mould with aubergine slices. Fill with layers of the tomato mixture, yogurt and aubergines, finishing with aubergines. Cover with foil and cook in the oven for 40-45 minutes, until tender. Leave for 10 minutes, then turn out on to a warmed serving dish. Heat any remaining tomato sauce with the stock and spoon around the charlotte.

Cook's Tip

Sliced or halved aubergines should always be sprinkled with salt and left to stand as this will draw out the bitter juices. Try filling aubergine shells with a similar tomato mixture, sprinkling lightly with cheese and baking.

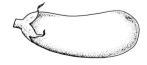

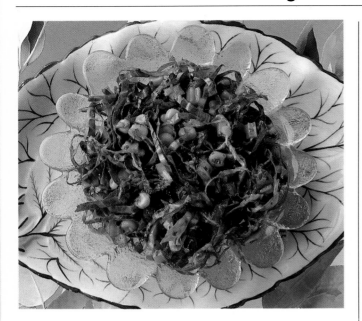

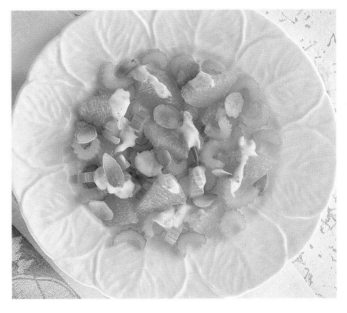

209 | Spring Green Salad

Preparation time
15 minutes, plus marinating

Serves 6

Calories
94 per portion

You will need
225 g/8 oz spring greens
3 tablespoons olive oil
2 teaspoons soy sauce
1 tablespoon lemon juice
2 garlic cloves, crushed
salt and pepper
3 celery sticks
½ x 200-g/7-oz can sweetcorn, drained
2 tablespoons chopped parsley

Shred the spring greens finely and place in a mixing bowl. Mix together the oil, soy sauce, lemon juice, garlic, and salt and pepper to taste and pour over the greens. Mix thoroughly and leave to marinate for 1 hour.

Slice the celery and add to the salad with the sweetcorn and parsley. Mix thoroughly, then transfer to a serving dish.

210 | Crisp Winter Salad

Preparation time
10 minutes

Cooking time
3 minutes

Serves 4

Calories
45 per portion

You will need
40 g/1½ oz flaked almonds
225 g/8 oz celery, thinly sliced
1 large orange, about 175 g/6 oz flesh, peeled, segmented and roughly chopped
150 ml/¼ pint natural low-fat yogurt
1 teaspoon ground coriander (optional)
½ teaspoon ground cumin or fennel seeds
pinch of salt (optional)

Place the almonds in an ungreased heavy-based frying pan over a low heat for 2-3 minutes, stirring until slightly browned.

Put half the almonds with the prepared celery and orange in a serving bowl and toss lightly.

Combine the yogurt, coriander (if using) and cumin or fennel seeds. Pour over the salad. Taste and add a little salt if necessary. Sprinkle the remaining almonds over the salad and serve.

Cook's Tip

You should aim to eat some raw vegetables every day as part of a healthy diet. Some people still associate salads with summer meals but equally appetizing mixtures can also be prepared in winter.

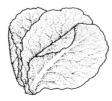

Cook's Tip

The crunchy combination of textures, sweetened with orange and spices, makes this salad a good addition to a winter menu. The yogurt blends perfectly with the orange to form a refreshing dressing.

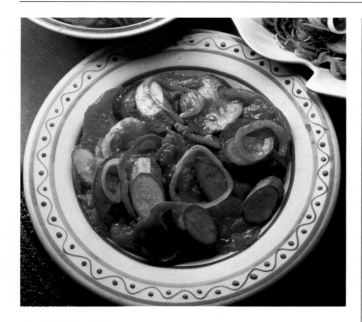

211 | *Poireaux Vinaigrette*

Preparation time
15 minutes, plus
chilling

Serves 4

Calories
133 per portion

You will need
6 leeks
1 tablespoon chopped capers

For the dressing
2 tablespoons lemon juice
3 tablespoons olive oil
1 teaspoon Meaux mustard
1 garlic clove, crushed
salt and pepper
1 tablespoon chopped parsley
1 tablespoon chopped chives

Slice the leeks very finely and arrange in a salad bowl.
   Put the dressing ingredients in a screw-topped jar and shake well. Pour over the leeks, add the capers and toss well. Chill for 1 hour before serving.

Cook's Tip

A good juicy lemon should yield about 3 tablespoons of juice. If you first warm the lemon in a cool oven, it will produce more juice. Try using other types of mustard in the dressing as a variation.

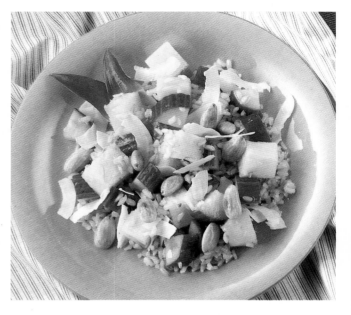

212 | *Tropical Salad*

Preparation time
15 minutes

Serves 4

Calories
357 per portion

You will need
275 g/10 oz long-grain brown rice,
   cooked
50 g/2 oz dried coconut flakes
½ cucumber, unpeeled and cut
   into 1 cm/½ inch cubes
1 small ripe pineapple, peeled,
   cored and cut into 2.5 cm/1 inch
   pieces
1 tablespoon olive oil
1 teaspoon lemon juice
salt and pepper

For the garnish
50 g/2 oz whole blanched
   almonds, toasted
pineapple leaves

Put the rice, coconut, cucumber and pineapple into a bowl. Add the oil and lemon juice and a little salt and pepper, taste and adjust the seasoning if necessary, then spoon into a serving dish.
   Scatter the almonds over the salad and garnish with the pineapple leaves.

Cook's Tip

Coconut flakes or slices are sold in many health food shops but unsweetened desiccated coconut can be substituted. If a fresh pineapple is not available, you can use a 400-g/14-oz can of pineapple in natural juice.

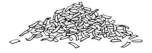

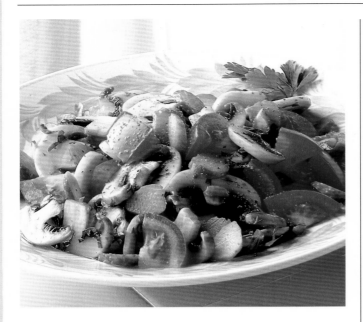

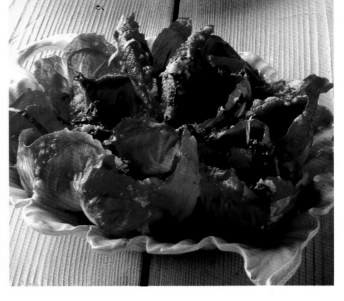

213 | *Mushroom Salad*

Preparation time
15 minutes, plus
standing

Serves 4

Calories
108 per portion

You will need
250 g/9 oz button mushrooms
juice of ½ lemon
2 tablespoons sliced gherkins
175 g/6 oz tomatoes, finely
   chopped
1 garlic clove, crushed with salt
1 parsley sprig, finely chopped
freshly ground black pepper
pinch of sugar
3 tablespoons olive oil

Trim the mushroom stalks level with the caps. Put into a sieve, rinse and drain thoroughly. Cut into thin slices, put into a bowl and sprinkle with the lemon juice. Add the gherkins and tomatoes and mix well to blend.

   To make the dressing, beat the garlic with the parsley, pepper to taste, sugar and oil. Pour over the mushroom salad and toss well to mix. Leave to marinate in the refrigerator for 10-15 minutes to allow the flavours to develop. Serve lightly chilled.

214 | *Radicchio with Garlic Dressing*

Preparation time
10 minutes, plus
standing

Serves 6

Calories
68 per portion

You will need
2 heads of radicchio
3 garlic cloves, finely chopped
1 tablespoon shredded basil
   leaves
salt and pepper
1 teaspoon grated Parmesan
   cheese
3 tablespoons olive oil
1 tablespoon wine vinegar

Remove the outer leaves from the radicchio and cut away the thick stems. Separate the leaves, tearing the larger leaves into pieces. Put in a sieve, rinse and drain thoroughly. Arrange in a salad bowl.

   To make the dressing, beat the garlic with the basil, salt and pepper to taste, cheese, oil and vinegar. Pour over the radicchio and toss lightly. Leave to stand for a few minutes before serving to allow the flavours to develop.

Cook's Tip

This piquant salad makes a delicious accompaniment to cold roast chicken. It can also be served as a starter or packed into a lidded plastic box for a picnic, preferably carried in a chill-bag.

Cook's Tip

This is a delicious simple salad which can be served as a starter or as an accompaniment. In Italy it is often eaten with plainly cooked veal escalopes, the red leaves providing an appetizing contrast to the pale meat.

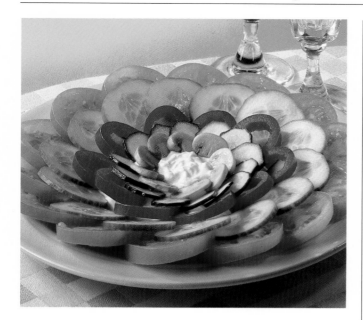

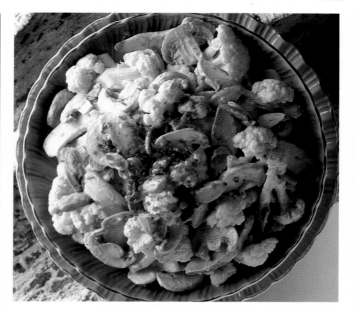

215 | Red and Green Salad

Preparation time
25 minutes, plus standing

Serves 4

Calories
220 per portion

You will need
225 g/8 oz courgettes, sliced
100 g/4 oz button mushrooms, thinly sliced
2 tablespoons snipped fresh chives
4 large tomatoes, thinly sliced
½ cucumber, thinly sliced
1 red pepper, seeded and thinly sliced into rings

For the dressing
4 tablespoons vegetable oil
2 tablespoons red wine vinegar
salt and pepper
pinch of mustard powder
5 tablespoons buttermilk, or natural low-fat yogurt
15 g/½ oz blue cheese, crumbled
50 g/2 oz Ricotta cheese, crumbled

Mix together the oil, vinegar, salt, pepper and mustard. Put the courgettes and the mushrooms in separate dishes and divide the dressing between them. Stir the chives into the courgettes. Set aside for at least 1 hour.

Arrange the tomatoes, cucumber and pepper in rings on a dish. Drain the courgettes, reserving the dressing, and make a ring with them. Drain the mushrooms, reserving the dressing, and arrange them in the centre.

Stir the buttermilk or yogurt into the dressing and stir in the cheeses. Spoon into the centre of the salad.

Cook's Tip

Ricotta is a low-fat Italian cheese which is made from the whey, not the curds, of cow's or goat's milk. It can be bought as a soft cheese or in a hardened form which is possible to grate.

216 | Cauliflower and Mushroom Salad

Preparation time
15 minutes, plus cooling

Cooking time
5 minutes

Serves 8

Calories
83 per portion

You will need
250 g/9 oz cauliflower, broken into florets
100 g/4 oz button mushrooms, sliced
1 avocado, halved, stoned, peeled and sliced
25 g/1 oz flaked almonds, toasted

For the dressing
150 ml/¼ pint natural low-fat yogurt
1 teaspoon lemon juice
1 garlic clove, crushed
paprika
chopped chives

Cook the cauliflower in boiling, salted water for 2 minutes; drain and leave to cool completely. Place in a bowl with the mushrooms, avocado and almonds.

Mix the dressing ingredients together, adding salt and paprika to taste. Pour over the vegetables and toss thoroughly. Transfer to a serving dish and sprinkle with the chives.

Cook's Tip

Avocados are high in calories so slimmers should not combine them with any dressing containing oil. Their creamy texture blends well with the cauliflower florets to make a light main course salad.

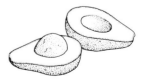

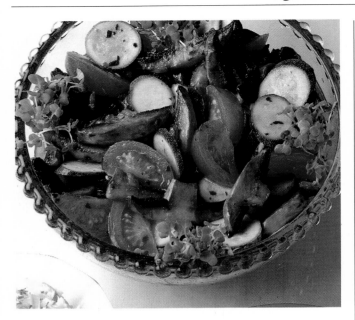

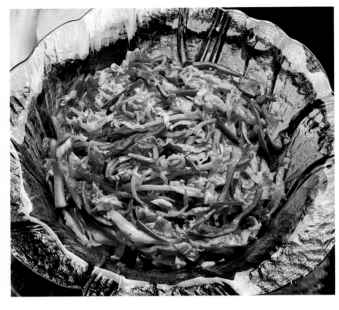

217 | Mushroom, Courgette and Tomato Salad

Preparation time
15 minutes

Serves 4

Calories
74 per portion

You will need
6 large mushrooms, sliced
4 courgettes, thinly sliced
4 tomatoes, peeled and quartered
1 teaspoon chopped fresh basil
1 bunch of cress, trimmed and
    divided into sprigs
3 tablespoons light French
    dressing (see Recipe 181)

Combine the mushrooms, courgettes and tomatoes in a salad bowl and sprinkle with the basil.

Arrange the sprigs of cress round the edge of the salad. Serve with the light French dressing.

218 | Chinese Salad

Preparation time
15 minutes

Serves 4

Calories
39 per portion

You will need
175 g/6 oz red cabbage, finely
    shredded
few Chinese leaves, shredded
100 g/4 oz bean sprouts, rinsed
2 celery sticks, chopped
5 cm/2 inch piece of cucumber,
    cut into strips

For the dressing
4 tablespoons natural low-fat
    yogurt
1 teaspoons soy sauce
salt and pepper

Put the red cabbage in a bowl and add the Chinese leaves, bean sprouts, celery and cucumber.

Mix together the dressing ingredients, with salt and pepper to taste, and add to the vegetables. Mix well and transfer to a serving bowl.

Cook's Tip

A combination of contrasting colours gives a salad visual appeal. Mushrooms, courgettes and tomatoes not only look good together, they also complement each other in taste. The salad could be bordered with watercress.

Cook's Tip

The addition of soy sauce gives a piquancy to the dressing. The Chinese leaves add both colour contrast and a crunchy texture to the salad.

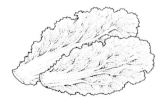

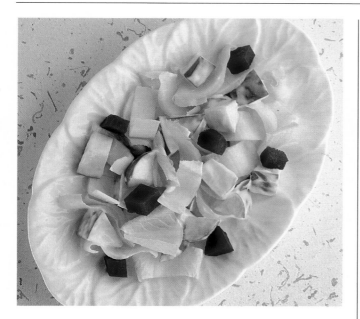

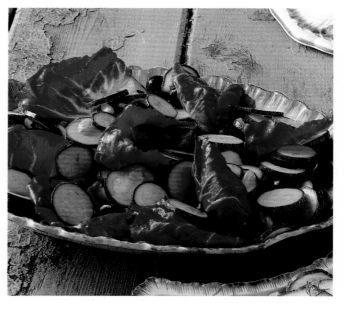

219 | Red and White Salad

Preparation time
15 minutes

Cooking time
50 minutes

Serves 4

Calories
88 per portion

You will need
225 g/8 oz fresh beetroot, scrubbed
225 g/8 oz eating apple, washed
about 2 tablespoons lemon juice
2 chicory heads, cut into 1 cm/
  ½ inch thick slices
150 ml/¼ pint natural low-fat
  yogurt or cultured buttermilk
¼ teaspoon pepper
½-1 teaspoon mild mustard
pinch of salt
2 teaspoons sunflower oil

Boil or steam the beetroot for about 50 minutes until tender. Drain and dice.

Quarter and core the apple, then cut into small cubes. Toss in the lemon juice immediately to avoid discolouration. Mix the apple with the chicory in a serving dish. Combine the yogurt or buttermilk, pepper, mustard, salt and oil in a jug. Spoon over the salad. Stir in the beetroot just before serving, as its colour will quickly stain the other salad ingredients.

220 | Courgette and Radicchio Salad

Preparation time
15 minutes, plus standing

Serves 6

Calories
95 per portion

You will need
4 tablespoons light French
  dressing (see Recipe 181)
1 garlic clove, crushed
250 g/9 oz courgettes, thinly
  sliced
1 head of radicchio
50 g/2 oz black olives, halved and
  stoned
1 tablespoon pine nuts
salt and pepper

Put the French dressing and garlic in a salad bowl. Add the sliced courgettes and toss well. Leave to stand for 30 minutes to allow the courgettes to absorb the flavour of the dressing.

Tear the radicchio leaves into manageable pieces and add to the courgettes and dressing with the black olives and pine nuts. Season with salt and pepper to taste. Toss the salad thoroughly before serving.

Cook's Tip

Cultured buttermilk is available in the dairy section of many large supermarkets. Sunflower oil is a useful all-purpose oil with a milder flavour than olive oil. Diced Chinese leaves may be used instead of the chicory.

Cook's Tip

Pine nuts are an important ingredient of vegetarian cooking. They are high in protein. They have long been used in Italian and French dishes. Always tear salad leaves rather than cut them.

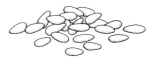

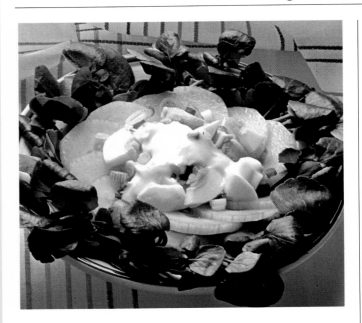

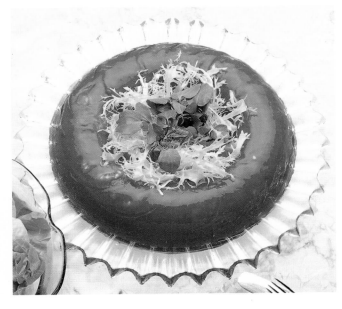

221 | Egg and Cucumber Salad

Preparation time
20 minutes

Serves 4

Calories
143 per portion

You will need
1 bunch of watercress
1 cucumber, peeled and sliced
4 hard-boiled eggs, finely chopped
1 bunch of spring onions, chopped

For the sauce
300 ml/½ pint natural low-fat
   yogurt
1 tablespoon lemon juice
1 teaspoon mustard powder
salt and pepper

Arrange the watercress in a serving dish and cover with the cucumber slices. Mix the chopped eggs and spring onions together and spoon into the centre.

To make the sauce, mix all the ingredients together. Pour over the salad and serve.

222 | Tomato Ring Salad

Preparation time
15 minutes, plus setting

Cooking time
5 minutes

Serves 4

Calories
53 per portion

You will need
4 tomatoes, skinned and sliced
600 ml/1 pint tomato juice
1 teaspoon Worcestershire sauce
salt and pepper
15 g/½ oz powdered gelatine
3 tablespoons water

For the garnish
endive leaves
watercress sprigs

Arrange the tomato slices in the base of a 900 ml/1½ pint ring mould. Pour the tomato juice into a small saucepan and bring to the boil. Reduce the heat and stir in the Worcestershire sauce with salt and pepper to taste.

Dissolve the gelatine with the water in a small bowl over a pan of gently simmering water. Combine with the tomato juice and pour into the mould. Allow to cool, then chill in the refrigerator for 3 hours, or until set.

To serve, dip the mould into hot water for a few seconds, then place a serving plate on top of the mould and invert with a sharp shake to unmould it. Fill the centre of the mould with endive leaves, top with watercress and serve chilled.

Cook's Tip

To avoid a black rim forming around the yolks of hard-boiled eggs, cook them for a maximum of 9 minutes and plunge into cold water immediately, tapping the shells as you do so. If you use a wet knife to slice hard-boiled eggs, the yolks will not crumble as you cut them.

Cook's Tip

For a complete light meal, fill the centre of the mould with cottage cheese mixed with finely chopped spring onion and fresh basil. Cheese always combines well with tomato.

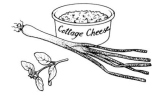

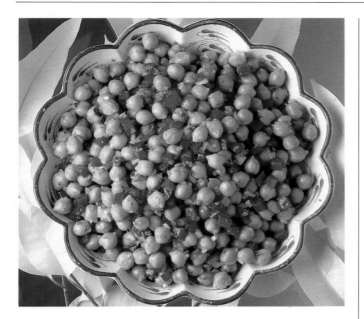

223 | Chick Pea Salad

Preparation time
*10 minutes, plus
soaking and cooling*

Cooking time
1½-2 hours

Serves 6

Calories
108 per portion

You will need
*250 g/9 oz chick peas, soaked
   overnight
salt
4 tablespoons light French
   dressing (see Recipe 181)
½ teaspoon ground ginger
1 small onion, chopped
1 red pepper, seeded and diced
2 tablespoons chopped parsley*

Drain the chick peas, put in a saucepan and cover with cold water. Bring to the boil and simmer for 1½-2 hours or until softened, adding a little salt towards the end of cooking.

Drain thoroughly and place in a bowl. Blend the French dressing with the ground ginger. Pour over the dressing and toss well while still warm. Leave to cool.

Add the remaining ingredients, toss thoroughly and transfer to a serving dish.

Cook's Tip

Although chick peas are also available canned, it is worth the effort of soaking the dried variety overnight as you then know no preservatives have been used in the liquor.

224 | Pasta and Bean Salad

Preparation time
*15 minutes, plus
cooling*

Cooking time
8-10 minutes

Serves 4

Calories
172 per portion

You will need
*2 tablespoons olive oil
3 tablespoons unsweetened
   orange juice
1 garlic clove, crushed
salt and pepper
2 tablespoons finely chopped
   parsley
175 g/6 oz wholemeal pasta
   shapes
175 g/6 oz cooked red kidney
   beans
50 g/2 oz soya bean sprouts
2 tablespoons natural low-fat
   yogurt
1 tablespoon chopped chives
75 g/3 oz alfalfa salad sprouts*

Mix the olive oil with the orange juice, garlic, salt and pepper to taste and the chopped parsley.

Cook the wholemeal pasta shapes in a large pan of boiling salted water until tender (8-10 minutes, depending on the size of the pasta shapes). Drain the pasta shapes thoroughly and stir into the orange and oil dressing while the pasta is still warm. Allow to cool.

Mix in the kidney beans and soya bean sprouts; stir in the yogurt and chives. Spoon the prepared salad on to a shallow serving dish and arrange the alfalfa salad sprouts around the edge. Serve as a complete light meal.

Cook's Tip

Soya bean and alfalfa salad sprouts can be grown at home. Soak 2 tablespoons of beans in water overnight, drain and put in a clean jam jar. Fill with water and leave in a dark place for 4 days, changing the water daily.

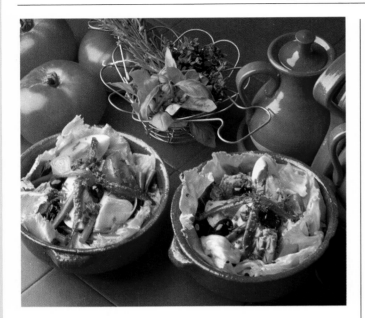

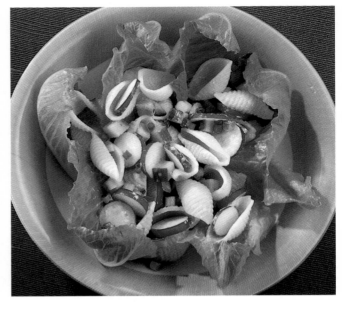

225 | *Salade Niçoise*

Preparation time
20 minutes

Serves 6

Calories
165 per portion

You will need
⅓ crisp lettuce
3 eggs, hard-boiled
1 x 400-g/14-oz can artichoke
    hearts
1 x 200-g/7-oz can tuna fish in
    brine, drained
1 x 50-g/2-oz can anchovy fillets,
    drained
250 g/9 oz tomatoes, peeled and
    quartered
150 g/5 oz French beans, cooked
8-10 black olives, stoned
1-2 teaspoons capers
1 tablespoon chopped parsley
4 tablespoons light French
    dressing (see Recipe 181)

Line a serving bowl with the lettuce.

Cut the eggs into quarters. Drain the artichoke hearts, tuna and anchovy fillets and arrange in the prepared bowl, together with the remaining salad ingredients.

Put the dressing ingredients in a screw-topped jar and shake well. Pour over the salad, toss well and serve immediately.

226 | *Pasta, Cucumber and Radish Salad*

Preparation time
20 minutes

Cooking time
10 minutes

Serves 4

Calories
66 per portion

You will need
100 g/4 oz pasta shapes
salt
175 g/6 oz radishes, trimmed,
    washed and sliced
½ cucumber, about 225 g//8 oz,
    unpeeled and diced
150 ml/¼ pint natural low-fat
    yogurt
freshly ground black pepper
1 cos lettuce, washed and dried
2 spring onions, trimmed, peeled
    and finely chopped, to garnish

Put the pasta into a large pan of boiling lightly salted water. Bring back to the boil and cook for about 10 minutes until 'al dente'. Rinse under cold running water and drain thoroughly.

Put the radishes and cucumber into a bowl and add the pasta. Stir in the yogurt adding plenty of black pepper and a little salt. Turn the pasta, radishes and cucumber over in the yogurt to coat thoroughly.

Arrange the lettuce leaves on a serving dish and spoon the salad into them. Garnish with the chopped spring onions.

Cook's Tip

Every cook along the Provençal coast has his or her own family recipe for Salade Niçoise. The locally caught tuna and anchovies are invariably included with the glossy black olives which grow in abundance.

Cook's Tip

For this main course salad, it is best not to peel the cucumber as its green skin looks so decorative. Choose from a wide variety of pasta shapes.

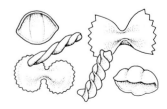

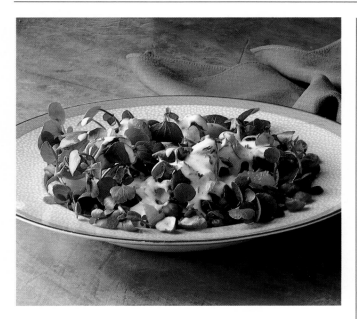

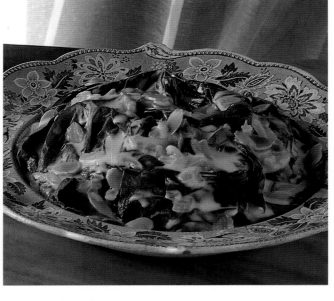

227 | Watercress with Orange and Nuts

Preparation time
15 minutes, plus
standing

Serves 4

Calories
63 per portion

You will need
1 bunch of watercress
1 large orange
1 tablespoon chopped hazelnuts
120 ml/4 fl oz natural low-fat
  yogurt
½ garlic clove, crushed with salt
pinch of sugar
2 teaspoons chopped parsley
freshly ground black pepper

Trim the watercress stems, sort the leaves, put in a sieve, rinse and drain thoroughly. Put in a large serving bowl.

Peel and segment the orange, removing all pith, then chop roughly. Add the orange and hazelnuts to the watercress.

To make the piquant dressing beat the yogurt with the garlic, sugar, parsley and pepper to taste. Pour over the watercress and toss well. Leave to stand for about 30 minutes before serving to allow the flavours to blend and develop.

228 | Spinach with Flaked Almonds

Preparation time
15 minutes

Cooking time
15-20 minutes

Serves 4

Calories
112 per portion

You will need
1 kg/2¼ lb leaf spinach
15 g/½ oz butter
½ onion, finely chopped
salt
grated nutmeg
3 tablespoons natural low-fat
  yogurt
40 g/1½ oz flaked almonds

Sort the spinach, put in a sieve, rinse and drain thoroughly. Tear the leaves into manageable pieces.

Melt the butter in a large pan, add the onion and cook for 2-3 minutes until softened. Add the spinach, a little at a time, turning it in the butter to coat. Season with salt and nutmeg to taste. Cover and cook over a low heat for 10-15 minutes, until tender, depending upon the thickness of the spinach leaves.

Stir the yogurt into the spinach mixture. Immediately remove the spinach from the heat and transfer to a warmed serving bowl. Add the flaked almonds to the butter remaining in the pan and fry, stirring, until golden. Fold the almonds into the spinach and serve immediately.

Cook's Tip

An attractive way of serving this salad as a starter is to fill the mixture into grapefruit or orange shells. These look even more attractive if you first vandyke the edges.

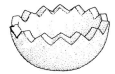

Cook's Tip

Other members of the spinach family such as spinach beet or orache may be cooked in the same way. If you add 2 egg yolks to the yogurt, this dish can be served as a light meal.

Desserts

The dessert course, usually high in calories, often proves an irresistible temptation to weight-watchers. The recipes in this chapter show how favourite desserts including fools and ice creams can still be enjoyed. Fruit is the obvious choice as a base for low-calorie desserts. Visually appealing and naturally sweet, it can be served in refreshing dishes such as Kiwi Fruit Salad and Stuffed Figs and combined with other ingredients to make both hot and cold desserts. Natural low-fat yogurt or sometimes smetana is used instead of cream in these recipes.

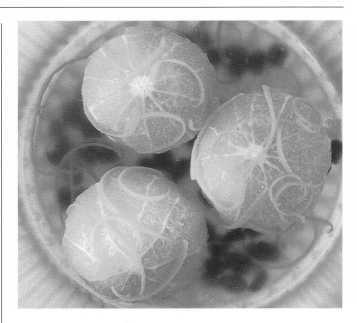

229 | Spiced Pears

Preparation time
20 minutes, plus cooling

Cooking time
15-20 minutes

Serves 4

Calories
82 per portion

You will need
4 large firm pears
½ lemon
16 cloves
½ cinnamon stick
300 ml/½ pint red wine
2 tablespoons redcurrant jelly
4 orange slices
4 small fresh bay leaves, to decorate

Peel the pears, leaving the stalks intact; rub them all over with the lemon half to prevent discolouration. Stud each pear with 4 cloves.

Stand the pears upright in a pan; add the cinnamon stick, wine and just sufficient water to cover the pears. Bring to the boil and simmer gently until the pears are tender. Leave to cool in the cooking liquid.

Put 2 tablespoons of the cooking liquid into a small pan with the redcurrant jelly; bubble briskly for about 1 minute until the jelly has dissolved.

Place an orange slice on each of four small plates; drain the pears with a slotted spoon, and sit one on top of each orange sliced. Spoon a little redcurrant glaze over each pear and decorate with a small bay leaf.

230 | Poached Oranges with Raisins

Preparation time
20 minutes, plus cooling

Cooking time
15 minutes

Serves 4

Calories
126 per portion

You will need
4 large oranges
300 ml/½ pint dry white wine
50 g/2 oz raisins
1 teaspoon powdered gelatine
2 tablespoons dry vermouth

Pare the rind from the oranges very thinly and cut it into fine matchstick strips. Put these into a saucepan with sufficient water to cover; bring to the boil and simmer for 4 minutes. Drain thoroughly and plunge the strips into a bowl of iced water.

Remove all the pith from the peeled oranges and put the fruit into a saucepan with the wine and raisins; simmer gently for 10 minutes, turning the oranges from time to time. Remove the oranges with a slotted spoon and place in a serving dish.

Dissolve the gelatine in the vermouth in a bowl over a saucepan of gently simmering water and stir into the cooking liquid; allow to cool and add half the orange rind strips. Spoon over the whole oranges, and scatter the remaining strips of rind around the oranges. Leave until completely cold.

Cook's Tip

This recipe is based on a dessert which was very popular in the early 18th century when spices were extensively used. Cinnamon stick is the dried bark of a species of laurel which flourishes in Sri Lanka.

Cook's Tip

The easiest way to remove any stubborn pieces of pith from an orange is with a clean razor blade. If you cannot find a suitable holder for the blade, try using a craft knife reserved for culinary use.

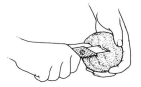

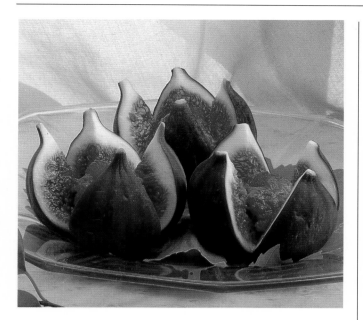

231 | Stuffed Figs

Preparation time
15 minutes

Serves 4

Calories
94 per portion

You will need
12 ripe fresh figs, preferably
  purple ones
3 tablespoons ground almonds
100 g/4 oz fresh raspberries
1 tablespoon honey
4 vine leaves, soaked in warm
  water and dried, to serve

Snip off any excess stalk from each fig; make a criss-cross cut down from the stalk end and carefully ease the cut open.

Mix the ground almonds with the fresh raspberries and honey. Place a vine leaf, spread out flat, on each serving plate; arrange three figs on top of each one, and fill with the raspberry and almond purée.

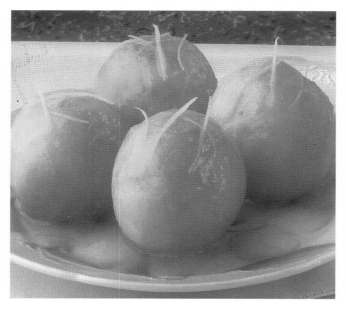

232 | Marinated Nectarines

Preparation time
25 minutes, plus
chilling

Serves 4

Calories
42 per portion

You will need
4 large ripe nectarines
1 lemon
1 large orange
200 ml/7 fl oz water
4 tablespoons dry vermouth

Nick the stalk end of each nectarine; plunge into a bowl of boiling water for 45 seconds, then slide off the skins. Pare the skin from the lemon and cut into matchstick strips. Squeeze the lemon juice into a large bowl and fill up with iced water. Put the prepared nectarines into the lemon water.

Peel the orange thinly, removing all the pith; chop the flesh into pieces, discarding any pips. Cut the orange peel into matchstick strips. Put the orange flesh into a liquidizer with the water and vermouth; blend until smooth.

Lift the nectarines out of the lemon water and drain. Put the nectarines into a shallow dish and spoon over the prepared orange and vermouth sauce. Cover and chill for 2 hours. (No longer, otherwise the nectarines are likely to discolour.)

Sprinkle with the strips of lemon and orange peel and serve immediately.

Cook's Tip

The stalk end of a ripe fig should feel slightly soft when pressed. If it is still hard, leave to ripen at room temperature. Fig or other decorative leaves can be used instead of vine leaves.

Cook's Tip

To remove the skin from either a nectarine or a peach, nick the stalk end with the tip of a sharp pointed knife and plunge the fruit into a bowl of boiling water for 45 seconds. The skin will then slide off effortlessly.

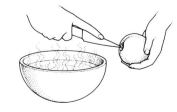

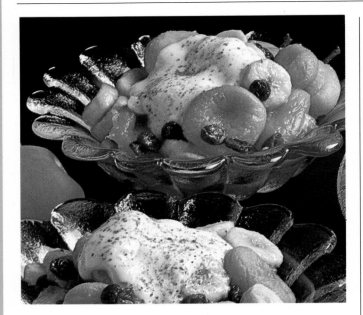

233 | *Apricot and Banana Compôte*

Preparation time
15 minutes, plus soaking and chilling

Serves 4

Calories
88 per portion

You will need
*100 g/4 oz dried apricots
2 bananas
2 teaspoons lemon juice
25 g/1 oz raisins
150 ml/¼ pint natural low-fat
    yogurt
few drops of artificial liquid
    sweetener (optional)
grated nutmeg*

Wash the apricots, put in a bowl and cover with cold water. Leave to soak overnight.

Slice the bananas and toss in the lemon juice. Place the apricots in a bowl with a little of the soaking liquid. Add the bananas and raisins, then divide the fruit between four glass serving dishes.

Sweeten the yogurt if preferred, spoon over the fruit and sprinkle with grated nutmeg. Chill before serving.

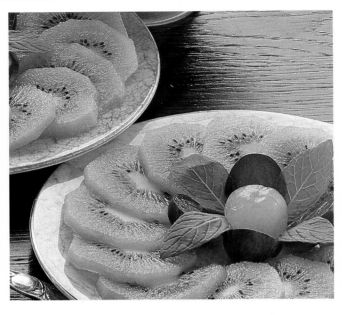

234 | *Kiwi Fruit Salad*

Preparation time
25 minutes, plus chilling

Serves 4

Calories
119 per portion

You will need
*8 kiwi fruit
4 plump green grapes
8 plump black grapes
2 tablespoons dry white wine
2 tablespoons unsweetened
    orange juice*

Peel the kiwi fruit and cut into thin slices; arrange these, overlapping, around the edges of four small plates. Skin the green grapes and halve the black ones.

Arrange the black grapes in the centre of each plate; place a whole green grape in the centre of this. Spoon the wine and the orange juice over and chill for 1 hour.

Cook's Tip

Keep bananas at room temperature until they are sufficiently ripe to use. Take care when removing a banana from the 'hand' not to loosen the skin of the adjoining fruit. You can save time by using no-soak apricots.

Cook's Tip

Egg-shaped kiwi fruit with its brown hairy skin is now available most of the year. The fruit is ripe when it feels soft to the touch. Peeled and cut into cubes or slices, it can be used in fruit salads and as decoration.

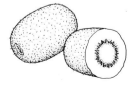

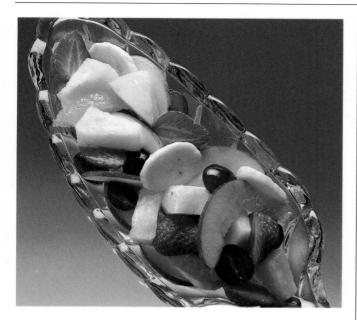

235 | Fresh Fruit Salad

Preparation time
25 minutes, plus chilling

Cooking time
4 minutes

Serves 8

Calories
83 per portion

You will need
2 tablespoons honey
120 ml/4 fl oz water
thinly pared rind and juice of
    1 lemon
1 red dessert apple, quartered and
    cored
1 pear, quartered and cored
1 banana
1 small pineapple
2 oranges
100 g/4 oz black grapes, halved
    and seeded
100 g/4 oz strawberries, sliced

Put the honey, water and lemon rind in a small saucepan. Bring to the boil, simmer for 2 minutes, then strain and leave to cool. Stir in the lemon juice.

Slice the apple, pear and banana into a bowl, pour over the lemon syrup and stir to coat the fruit. Peel the pineapple with a sharp knife and cut the flesh into sections, discarding the central core. Peel the oranges, removing all pith, and divide into two segments. Add to the bowl with the pineapple, grapes and strawberries and mix.

Turn into a glass dish and chill until required.

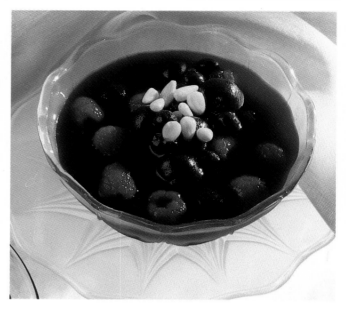

236 | Cassis Fruit Salad

Preparation time
30 minutes, plus chilling

Serves 6

Calories
73 per portion

You will need
3 tablespoons unsweetened
    orange juice
4 tablespoons crème de cassis
2 tablespoons clear honey
450 g/1 lb black dessert cherries,
    stoned
225 g/8 oz ripe blackcurrants,
    trimmed and 'tailed'
225 g/8 oz loganberries or
    raspberries, hulled
2 tablespoons pine nuts

Mix together the orange juice, crème de cassis and honey and stir until the honey has dissolved. Mix the cherries, blackcurrants and berries. Pour over the cassis mixture, stir well, cover and chill for at least 3 hours. Some of the juice will be drawn from the fruit to make a tangy dressing.

Scatter on the pine nuts just before serving. Serve chilled, with natural low-fat yogurt.

Cook's Tip

It is essential to use fresh strawberries in this fruit salad but canned pineapple could be substituted for fresh if this is not available. Choose a variety which is canned in natural juice, not syrup.

Cook's Tip

In the soft fruit season you will find many PYO (pick your own) signs on country roads. Take advantage of such opportunities to obtain high quality fruit at lower prices than charged in a shop.

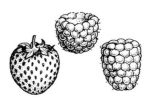

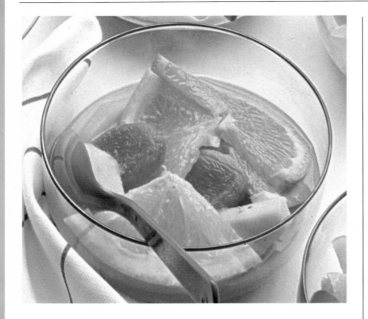

237 | Baked Fruit Salad

Preparation time
10 minutes

Cooking time
20 minutes

Oven temperature
200°C, 400°F, gas 6

Serves 4

Calories
79 per portion

You will need
1 grapefruit
2 oranges
1 eating apple, sliced
8 dried apricot halves
300 ml/½ pint unsweetened
    orange juice

Slice the grapefruit and oranges, leaving on the peel. Put the grapefruit, orange and apple slices in a casserole with the apricots. Use the ends of the oranges and grapefruit to cover the top.

Pour in the orange juice and cover with a lid or foil. Bake in the oven for about 20 minutes until all the fruit is soft. Serve hot or cold.

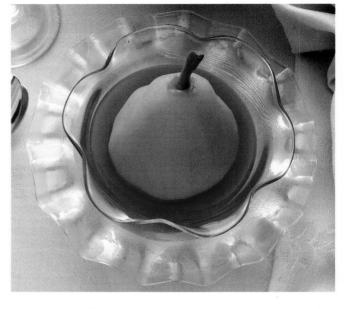

238 | Rosy Pears

Preparation time
10 minutes

Cooking time
30 minutes

Oven temperature
200°C, 400°F, gas 6

Serves 4

Calories
83 per portion

You will need
4 large firm pears, peeled
250 ml/8 fl oz unsweetened
    orange juice
120 ml/4 fl oz red wine
20-30 cardamom seeds, crushed
artificial liquid sweetener, to taste

Put the pears in an ovenproof dish and pour on the orange juice and red wine with the cardamom seeds. Bake in the oven for about 30 minutes until tender.

Taste the juice for sweetness and, if liked, add sweetener. Serve hot or chilled with the strained sauce.

Cook's Tip

A suitable apple to use in this fruit salad is a Cox's Orange Pippin. Served hot, this nutritious dish is a healthy way to start breakfast on a cold morning. It is equally good served cold.

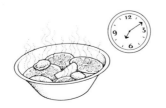

Cook's Tip

Cardamom seeds are strongly aromatic and can be used to flavour both sweet and savoury dishes. Choose a light red wine to cook the pears and tint them a delicate pink.

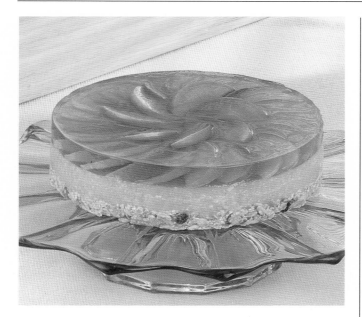

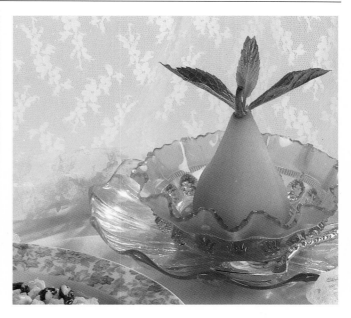

239 | Apple Gâteau

Preparation time
20 minutes, plus
chilling

Cooking time
20 minutes

Oven temperature
190°C, 375°F, gas 5

Serves 4

Calories
143 per portion

You will need
2 teaspoons powdered gelatine
2 tablespoons water
450 g/1 lb cooking apples, peeled,
   cored and sliced
grated rind and juice of ½ lemon
artificial sweetener, to taste
1 egg yolk
4 tablespoons muesli cereal
25 g/1 oz low-fat spread
2 dessert apples, sliced
150 ml/¼ pint apple juice

Dissolve 1 teaspoon of the gelatine in the water in a bowl over a saucepan of gently simmering water.

Poach the cooking apples with the lemon rind and juice and a few tablespoons of water until tender. Add sweetener to taste and beat in the egg yolk. Stir in the gelatine.

Bake the muesli in the oven for 8 minutes. Mix with the low-fat spread while still hot. Spread the muesli over the base of a loose-bottomed 18 cm/7 inch cake tin. Chill for 30 minutes.

Poach the dessert apple slices gently in the apple juice for about 3 minutes; remove carefully and drain on absorbent kitchen paper.

Dissolve the remaining gelatine in 2 tablespoons of the apple juice in a bowl over a saucepan of gently simmering water. Stir in the remaining apple juice.

Spread the apple purée over the muesli base; arrange the apple slices on top. Spoon over the apple juice glaze and chill for 4 hours.

Cook's Tip

*Most proprietary brands of
muesli contain some form of
sweetening. It is therefore
advisable to make your own
mixture by combining rolled
oats, wheat flakes, wheat
germ, a few chopped nuts and
some raisins.*

240 | Baked Cranberry Pears

Preparation time
25 minutes

Cooking time
40 minutes

Oven temperature
200°C, 400°F, gas 6

Serves 4

Calories
134 per portion

You will need
4 large, ripe dessert pears, peeled
   but with the stalks in place
225 g/8 oz cranberries, thawed, if
   frozen
1 tablespoon chopped hazelnuts
3 tablespoons clear honey
150 ml/¼ pint dry white wine
few drops of red food colouring
mint sprigs, to decorate

Working from the base and using a small teaspoon, scoop out the pear cores. Chop 2 tablespoons of the cranberries and mix with the nuts and 1 tablespoon of the honey. Press the mixture into the pear cavities.

Put the remaining cranberries, honey, wine and a few drops of red food colouring in a flameproof dish and bring to the boil over a moderate heat. Simmer for 5 minutes. Stand the pears upright in the dish and spoon the wine over them.

Cover the dish lightly with foil and cook in the oven for 30 minutes, basting the pears with the wine once or twice. Decorate each pear with a sprig of mint and serve hot or cold.

Cook's Tip

*The colour of honey depends
on the type of flowers from
which the bees have collected
nectar. For example, acacia
honey is a very pale golden
colour whereas heather honey
is much darker.*

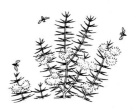

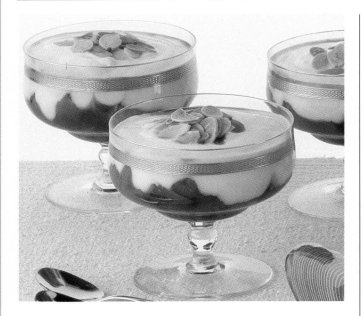

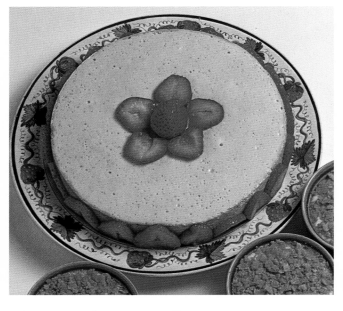

241 | *Rhubarb and Raspberry Layer*

Preparation time
15 minutes, plus
chilling

Cooking time
10-15 minutes

Serves 4

Calories
161 per portion

You will need
450 g/1 lb fresh rhubarb
225 g/8 oz fresh or frozen
   raspberries
50 g/2 oz soft brown sugar
225 g/8 oz low-fat soft cheese
150 ml/¼ pint natural low-fat
   yogurt
fresh raspberries or toasted
   almonds, to decorate

Wash and chop the rhubarb and put in a pan with the raspberries and sugar. Simmer for 10-15 minutes, until soft.

Blend in the cheese with the yogurt. Layer the fruit and yogurt mixture in four individual glass dishes. Chill for 2 hours. Decorate the pudding with raspberries or with toasted almonds before serving.

242 | *Strawberry Mould*

Preparation time
20 minutes, plus
setting

Serves 6

Calories
68 per portion

You will need
225 g/8 oz cottage cheese, sieved
150 ml/¼ pint natural low-fat
   yogurt
250 g/9 oz strawberries, puréed
3 teaspoons powdered gelatine
3 tablespoons water
3-4 drops of artificial liquid
   sweetener
2 egg whites
100 g/4 oz fresh sliced
   strawberries, to decorate

Mix together the cottage cheese, yogurt and strawberry purée.

Dissolve the gelatine in the water in a bowl over a pan of gently simmering water. Cool, then fold into the cheese mixture with sweetener to taste.

Whisk the egg whites until stiff and fold into the mixture. Pour into a 20 cm/8 inch loose-bottomed flan tin. Chill until set (about 3 hours).

Remove from the tin, place on a serving plate and decorate with the sliced strawberries.

Cook's Tip

**Use a pair of sharp kitchen
scissors to cut the rhubarb
into even lengths. It is easier
to avoid having any loose
stringy bits when the rhubarb
is cut in this way.**

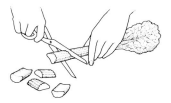

Cook's Tip

**By sieving cottage cheese you
can achieve a similar texture
to curd cheese but with
significantly fewer calories.
First press out and discard any
whey with the back of a
wooden spoon.**

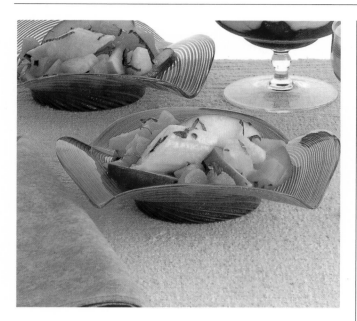

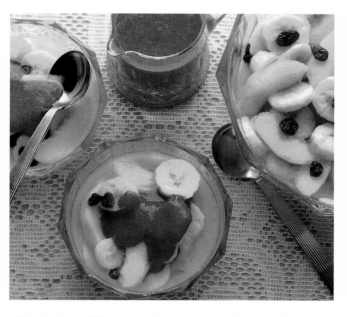

243 | Honey Mint Fruit

Preparation time
20 minutes, plus
chilling

Cooking time
20-25 minutes

Oven temperature
180°C, 350°F, gas 4

Serves 4

Calories
113 per portion

You will need
8 dried apricots, chopped
2 dessert pears, peeled, cored
    and chopped
2 bananas, thickly sliced
2 red dessert apples, cored and
    sliced
2 pineapple rings, chopped
2 teaspoons lemon juice
2 tablespoons dry cider
2 teaspoons clear honey
12 mint leaves, finely chopped, or
    ½ teaspoon dried mint

Put all the fruit in a 1.2 litre/2 pint heatproof dish.

Mix together the lemon juice, cider and honey, then pour over the fruit. Stir in the mint and mix well. Cover and cook in the oven for 20-25 minutes. Chill slightly, then serve.

244 | Raspberry Fruit Cocktail

Preparation time
15 minutes, plus
standing and chilling

Serves 4

Calories
83 per portion

You will need
2 bananas
2 teaspoons lemon juice
2 peaches
25 g/1 oz raisins
4 tablespoons fresh orange juice
150 g/5 oz raspberries
a pinch of nutmeg

Peel and slice the bananas and brush the slices with lemon juice to prevent discolouration. Put in a bowl. Peel, stone and slice the peaches, then add to the bananas with the raisins. Add the orange juice and stir gently to mix. Leave for 30 minutes for the flavours to blend.

Divide the fruit between four individual glasses or dessert bowls.

Purée the raspberries by rubbing them through a sieve. Spoon a portion of raspberry purée over each serving of fruit to decorate and sprinkle with a pinch of nutmeg. Chill until ready to serve.

Cook's Tip

Mint can be grown very successfully in a large pot either on a window sill or in the garden where it is more easily controlled this way. Fresh mint leaves taste very much nicer than dried.

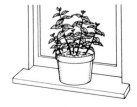

Cook's Tip

Most supermarkets now sell freshly squeezed orange juice in 500 ml/18 fl oz and 1 litre/ 1¾ pint bottles. It is much quicker to use this than to squeeze the fruit yourself. The juice can be stored in the refrigerator for several days.

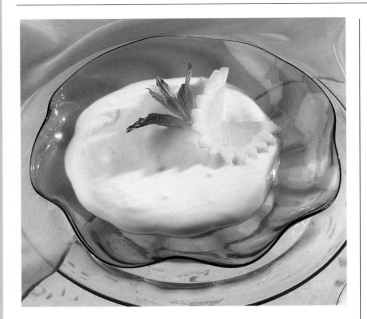

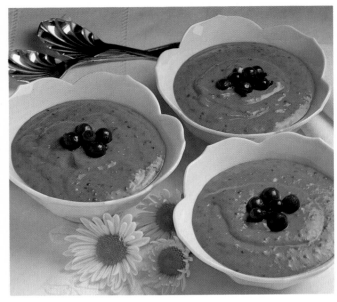

245 | Lemon Yogurt Syllabub

Preparation time
15 minutes, plus chilling

Serves 4

Calories
144 per portion

You will need
450 ml/¾ pint thick yogurt
1 tablespoon clear honey
grated rind of 1 lemon
juice of 2 lemons
2 tablespoons dry sherry
fresh fruit, to decorate

Whisk the yogurt in a bowl, then beat in the honey and lemon rind. Gradually add the lemon juice and sherry, stirring all the time.

Divide the mixture between four individual serving glasses. This syllabub is particularly delicious if served topped with a few fresh raspberries, strawberries or blackberries. Alternatively, decorate each glass with a thin slice of lemon and a sprig of mint. Serve chilled.

246 | Blackcurrant Fool

Preparation time
20 minutes, plus chilling

Cooking time
15 minutes

Serves 4

Calories
54 per portion

You will need
1 tablespoon cornflour
300 ml/½ pint skimmed milk
few drops of artificial liquid sweetener
300 g/10 oz blackcurrants
1 tablespoon water
150 ml/¼ pint natural low-fat yogurt
few blackcurrants, to decorate

Blend the cornflour with a little of the milk. Heat the remaining milk and stir into the cornflour mixture, then return to the saucepan. Heat, stirring continuously until the mixture thickens. Cook for 1 minute. Add sweetener to taste and leave to cool.

Trim and wash the blackcurrants, then put in a pan with the water. Cook gently until the fruit is soft. Add sweetener to taste and leave to cool. Purée the fruit in a blender or rub through a sieve.

Add the fruit purée and yogurt to the sauce and whisk until well blended. Spoon into four individual serving dishes and decorate with blackcurrants. Chill before serving.

Cook's Tip

Greek yogurt has quite a high fat content but you can make a yogurt of comparable consistency from skimmed long-life milk. This has already been heat-treated so it is not necessary to scald it before adding the culture. By adding skimmed milk powder to the milk you can make even thicker yogurt.

Cook's Tip

If possible, use a blender to purée the blackcurrants rather than rubbing the fruit through a sieve as this reduces the fibre content which is mostly in the seeds. This means that the blackcurrants need to be prepared carefully.

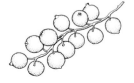

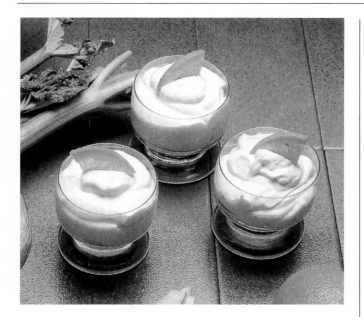

247 | Orange Pots

Preparation time
15 minutes, plus chilling

Cooking time
5 minutes

Serves 4

Calories
29 per portion

You will need
4 teaspoons powdered gelatine
3 tablespoons fresh orange juice
350 g/12 oz curd cheese
3 tablespoons lemon juice
3 tablespoons skimmed milk
artificial liquid sweetener, to taste
4 orange slices

Dissolve the gelatine in the orange juice in a bowl over a saucepan of gently simmering water.

Blend the gelatine mixture with the remaining ingredients, adding sweetener to taste. Spoon into individual serving dishes and top each with a slice of orange.

Cook's Tip

This mixture makes an excellent dessert for a celebration picnic. Fill into individual plastic containers, top with a slice of orange and cover with a lid or cling film. Transport to the picnic in a chill-bag.

248 | Blackberry Surprise

Preparation time
20 minutes, plus chilling

Cooking time
7 minutes

Serves 6

Calories
134 per portion

You will need
450 g/1 lb blackberries
3 teaspoons clear honey
1 tablespoon lemon juice
2 teaspoons powdered gelatine
175 g/6 oz natural low-fat yogurt
4 Petit Suisse cheeses
2 egg whites
2 tablespoons port
1 tablespoon hazelnuts
2 slivers lemon rind, chopped

Place half the blackberries in a heavy-based saucepan over a gentle heat and stir until softened. Stir in 2 teaspoons of the honey. Remove from the heat, add the lemon juice and sprinkle in the gelatine, stirring well to dissolve. Rub through a sieve, then leave the mixture to cool and thicken.

Combine the yogurt and Petit Suisse cheeses and stir in the cooled blackberry purée. Whip the egg whites until stiff and fold in.

Reserve a few whole blackberries for decoration. Divide the remainder between six tall wineglasses and pour 1 teaspoon of port into each. Top up with the blackberry mixture and chill.

Just before serving, dry-fry the hazelnuts with the lemon rind. When evenly coloured, chop them and sprinkle a little over each glass. Decorate with the remaining berries and honey.

Cook's Tip

Both cultivated and wild blackberries freeze extremely well. Just put the freshly picked fruit in a rigid plastic container and freeze. If you happen to pick some more berries later, these can be added to the others.

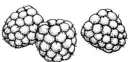

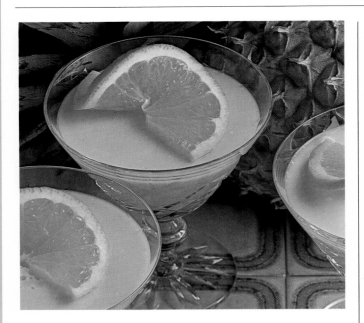

249 | Orange and Pineapple Jelly

Preparation time
10 minutes, plus
setting

Cooking time
3 minutes

Serves 4

Calories
109 per portion

You will need
150 ml/¼ pint water
1 packet orange jelly
200 ml/7 fl oz unsweetened
   pineapple juice
150 ml/¼ pint natural low-fat
   yogurt
orange twists, to decorate

Heat the water in a saucepan and add the jelly. Stir until dissolved, then add the pineapple juice. Pour into a bowl and place in the refrigerator until just beginning to set.

Whisk in the yogurt until well blended, then pour into four glass serving dishes. Leave until set, then decorate with orange twists.

Cook's Tip

Instead of a packet of orange jelly, you can use powdered gelatine with equal quantities of unsweetened orange and pineapple juices. Vegetarians can use agar in similar proportions as a substitute for gelatine.

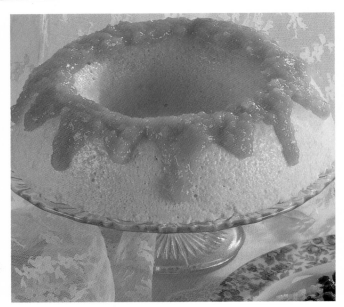

250 | Apple Ring with Apricot Sauce

Preparation time
30 minutes, plus
soaking and setting

Cooking time
30 minutes

Serves 6

Calories
94 per portion

You will need
450 g/1 lb cooking apples, peeled,
   cored and chopped
150 ml/¼ pint water
grated rind and juice of 1 lemon
2 cloves
25 g/1 oz powdered gelatine
2 eggs, separated
40 g/1 ½ oz muscovado sugar
150 ml/¼ pint low-fat yogurt

For the sauce
100 g/4 oz dried apricots
300 ml/½ pint water
rind and juice of ½ lemon
½ cinnamon stick
1 clove

Place the apples in a saucepan with the water, lemon rind and cloves. Bring to the boil and simmer for about 10 minutes. Discard the cloves.

Dissolve the gelatine in the lemon juice in a bowl over a saucepan of gently simmering water. Add to the apple mixture and blend in a liquidizer. Set aside to cool.

Whisk the egg yolks with the sugar until light and fluffy. Stir into the apple purée with the yogurt. Whisk the egg whites until stiff and fold into the purée.

Rinse a 1.2 litre/2 pint ring mould with cold water. Pour in the apple mixture and chill for 3 hours. Meanwhile make the sauce (see Cook's Tip).

Turn the apple mould on to a serving dish, drizzle a little of the sauce over it and serve the remainder separately.

Cook's Tip

To make the sauce, soak the apricots in the water for 2 hours. Put in a saucepan, add the lemon rind, lemon juice, cinnamon and clove, bring to the boil and simmer for 20 minutes. Remove the spices and purée the apricots.

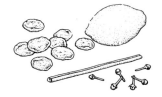

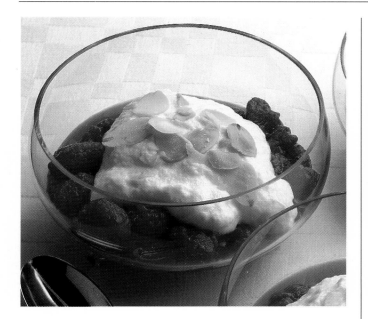

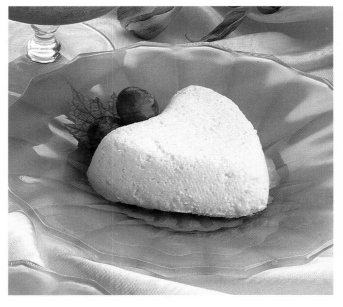

251 | Raspberry Chantilly

Preparation time
15 minutes, plus
chilling

Serves 4

Calories
102 per portion

You will need
450 g/1 lb raspberries, hulled
1 tablespoon Grand Marnier
2 egg whites
150 g/5 oz quark
grated rind of ½ orange
1 tablespoon caster sugar
25 g/1 oz toasted flaked almonds,
to decorate

Divide the raspberries equally among four individual glasses or dessert bowls, then spoon over the Grand Marnier. Cover with cling film and chill until ready to serve.

Whisk the egg whites stiffly, then gently fold in the quark, orange rind and sugar. Spoon the mixture over the raspberries and decorate with the almonds. Serve immediately.

252 | Curd Cheese Hearts

Preparation time
20 minutes, plus
draining

Serves 4

Calories
88 per portion

You will need
225 g/8 oz cottage cheese, sieved
artificial liquid sweetener, to taste
150 ml/¼ pint natural low-fat
yogurt
2 egg whites
1 tablespoon brandy

For the decoration
tiny fresh vine leaves (if available)
small clusters of black grapes

Mix the cottage cheese with a little sweetener to taste (if you do not have a very sweet tooth, this may not be necessary); blend in the yogurt. Whisk the egg whites until stiff but not dry; fold lightly but thoroughly into the cheese mixture together with the brandy.

Line four small perforated heart-shaped moulds with clean muslin; spoon the cheese mixture into the lined moulds and cover with another layer of muslin. Stand the moulds on a baking tray with a rim, and chill for 6-8 hours; the excess liquid should have drained away from the cheese, and the moulds should be firm enough to turn out.

Unmould the hearts and decorate with vine leaves and clusters of grapes.

Cook's Tip

Quark is a soft white cheese made from semi-skimmed milk. It does not contain salt. The fat content can vary quite considerably so it is advisable to check the label carefully before buying.

Cook's Tip

If you do not have the traditional moulds, make holes in yogurt or cottage cheese cartons and use these in the same way. Rinse the muslin after use in tepid water containing some bicarbonate of soda before washing.

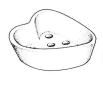

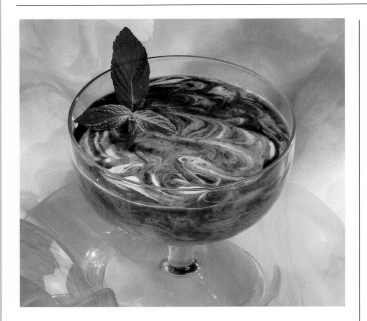

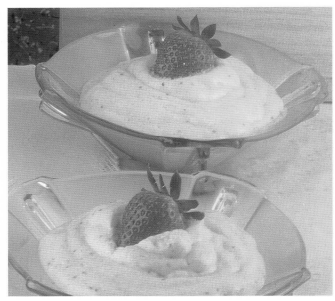

253 | Blueberry Creams

Preparation time
20 minutes, plus
chilling

Cooking time
20 minutes

Serves 4

Calories
82 per portion

You will need
3 tablespoons clear honey
2 tablespoons orange juice
1½ teaspoons grated orange rind
450 g/1 lb blueberries
3 tablespoons wholemeal flour
150 ml/¼ pint natural low-fat
   yogurt
4 small mint sprigs, to decorate

Put the honey, orange juice and orange rind into a saucepan and stir over a low heat until the honey has melted. Add the blueberries and simmer for 10 minutes, or until the fruit is tender. Purée the fruit and juice in a liquidizer, or rub them through a sieve.

Stir a little of the purée into the flour to make a smooth paste. Stir in the remaining purée, return it to the pan and stir over a medium heat until the purée thickens. Simmer for 3 minutes. Cool slightly, then divide the fruit purée between four individual serving glasses and chill for 2 hours.

Stir the yogurt through the blueberry purée and decorate with mint sprigs. Serve chilled.

254 | Strawberry and Orange Chiffon

Preparation time
35-40 minutes, plus
chilling

Serves 4

Calories
90 per portion

You will need
350 g/12 oz ripe strawberries
6 tablespoons orange juice
finely grated rind of ½ orange
1 tablespoon honey
2 eggs, separated
2 teaspoons powdered gelatine
2 tablespoons water
4 tablespoons natural low-fat
   yogurt

Reserve four whole strawberries for decoration. Put the remaining strawberries into a liquidizer and blend until smooth.

Put the orange juice and rind, honey and egg yolks into a bowl; whisk until thick, light and creamy.

Dissolve the gelatine in the water in a bowl over a saucepan of slightly simmering water.

Combine the strawberry purée and whisked egg yolk mixture, then stir in the dissolved gelatine and the yogurt. Leave until the mixture is about to set. Then whisk the egg whites until stiff but not dry and fold lightly but thoroughly into the strawberry mixture.

Spoon into individual glass dessert dishes and chill for 3 hours. Decorate each dessert with one of the reserved whole strawberries and serve.

Cook's Tip

Blueberries are known by a variety of other names including bilberries and whinberries in different parts of Britain. The fruit purée freezes well if packed in a tightly covered container.

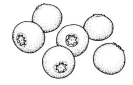

Cook's Tip

It is not necessary to use large, perfect strawberries for this dessert. Slightly over-ripe berries or the smaller ones known as jamming strawberries are perfectly suitable. If you do not have a sweet tooth, omit the honey.

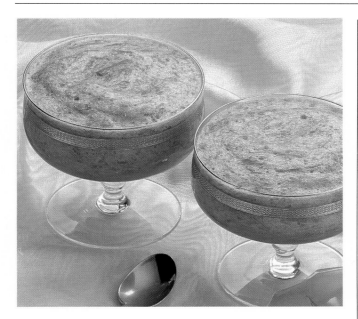

255 | Rhubarb and Ginger Flummery

Preparation time
20 minutes, plus setting

Cooking time
12 minutes

Serves 4

Calories
65 per portion

You will need
450 g/1 lb rhubarb, trimmed and chopped into rough lengths
grated rind and juice of ½ orange
¼ teaspoon ground ginger
3 tablespoons clear honey
2 teaspoons powdered gelatine
2 tablespoons water
2 egg whites

Put the rhubarb into a saucepan with the orange rind and juice, ginger and honey. Simmer gently until the fruit is quite soft. Dissolve the gelatine in the water in a bowl over a saucepan of gently simmering water and add to the cooked rhubarb. Beat until smooth. Cool the rhubarb mixture until it is just on the point of setting.

Whisk the egg whites until stiff but not dry; fold lightly but thoroughly into the semi-set rhubarb mixture. Spoon into tall stemmed glasses. Chill until set.

256 | Orange Honey Fluff

Preparation time
10 minutes, plus chilling

Serves 4

Calories
65 per portion

You will need
25 g/1 oz honey
grated rind and juice of 1 orange
2 teaspoons lemon juice
300 ml/½ pint natural low-fat yogurt
2 egg whites
few strips of orange rind, to decorate

Blend the honey with the orange and lemon juice. Stir in the grated orange rind and yogurt.

Whisk the egg whites until stiff and fold into the mixture. Spoon into four sundae dishes and decorate with the orange rind. Serve lightly chilled. Do not leave in the refrigerator for more than 1 hour or the mixture will start to separate.

Cook's Tip

Rhubarb is the first home-grown fruit of the season to appear in the shops. Choose slender crisp stems for the best flavour. As the leaves are inedible, these should be carefully cut away with any portion of the crown or root.

Cook's Tip

Remember to take the egg whites out of the refrigerator 30 minutes before you whisk them. This will help to increase their bulk. Eggs should be stored with the pointed ends downwards to keep them fresh longer.

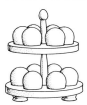

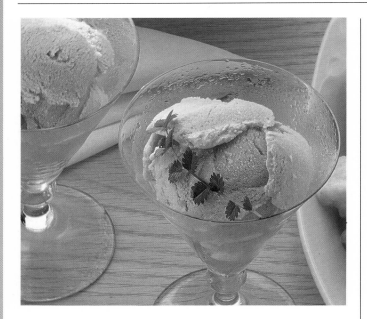

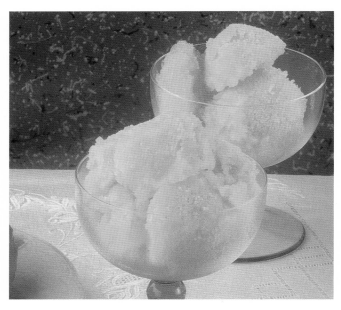

257 | Raspberry and Yogurt Ice Cream

Preparation time
10 minutes, plus
freezing

Serves 4

Calories
206 per portion

You will need
225 g/8 oz fresh raspberries
50 g/2 oz icing sugar
2 tablespoons clear honey
2 tablespoons lemon juice
900 ml/1½ pints natural low-fat
   yogurt
sprigs of fresh salad burnet (if
   available), to decorate

If freezing the ice cream in the refrigerator set at its lowest temperature. Liquidize the raspberries, then rub them through a sieve. Add all the other ingredients, stir well and freeze as fast as possible either in the freezing compartment of the refrigerator or in the freezer. Scoop the ice cream into glasses and decorate each serving with a sprig of salad burnet.

258 | Peach Granita

Preparation time
15 minutes, plus
freezing

Cooking time
6 minutes

Serves 4

Calories
92 per portion

You will need
350 g/12 oz fresh ripe peaches
150 ml/¼ pint dry white wine
150 ml/¼ pint fresh orange juice
2 egg whites

Remove the skin from each peach (see Recipe 232). Halve the fruit, removing the stones, and chop the flesh roughly.

Put the peach flesh into a saucepan with the white wine and orange juice. Simmer gently for 5 minutes. Then blend the peaches and the liquid in a liquidizer until smooth. Leave to cool. Put the mixture into a shallow container; freeze until the granita is 'slushy' around the edges, then tip into a bowl and break up the ice crystals. Whisk the egg whites until stiff but not dry; fold lightly but thoroughly into the partly-frozen granita. Return to the container and re-freeze for 2-3 hours until firm.

Cook's Tip

The young leaves of garden or salad burnet taste and smell rather like cucumber which is why they were once much used in wine cups. Another species of burnet grows wild in chalky districts of Britain.

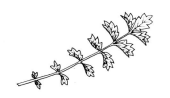

Cook's Tip

This type of iced dessert is very refreshing on a hot summer day. The peaches and fresh orange juice provide enough natural sweetness to make it unnecessary to use any artificial sweetener.

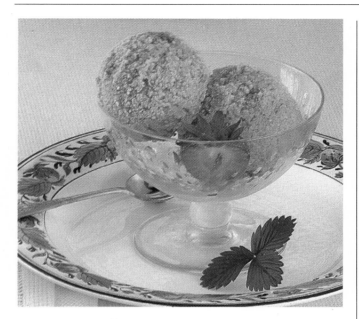

259 | Whole Strawberry Ice Cream

Preparation time
15 minutes, plus
freezing

Serves 4

Calories
79 per portion

You will need
3 egg yolks
1 tablespoon redcurrant jelly
1 tablespoon red vermouth
300 ml/½ pint natural low-fat
   yogurt
350 g/12 oz ripe strawberries,
   hulled
8 strawberries with stalks, halved,
   to decorate

Put the egg yolks into a blender or food processor with the redcurrant jelly, vermouth, yogurt and half the strawberries; blend until smooth. Transfer the mixture to a shallow container, and freeze until the ice cream starts to harden around the edges.

Tip the ice cream into a bowl and beat to break up the ice crystals. Chop the remaining strawberries and mix into the semi-set ice cream. Return to the container and freeze until quite firm. Scoop the ice cream into stemmed glasses and decorate each one with strawberry halves.

260 | Coffee Sorbet

Preparation time
5 minutes, plus
freezing

Serves 4

Calories
99 per portion

You will need
600 ml/1 pint natural low-fat
   yogurt
4 tablespoons skimmed milk
   powder
4 teaspoons instant coffee
   powder or granules
artificial liquid sweetener, to taste

Mix the yogurt, skimmed milk powder and instant coffee together. Add artificial sweetener to taste and stir well.

Pour into a shallow dish and freeze for 2-3 hours. Stir occasionally, mixing the frozen edges to the centre. The mixture should be eaten when quite soft.

Cook's Tip

Strawberries should be spread out on a plate and kept in the refrigerator or a cool place if not being eaten immediately. The fruit should always be washed before it is hulled to prevent the juice seeping.

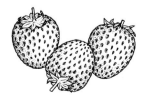

Cook's Tip

The skimmed milk powder gives a deliciously smooth texture to the sorbet and helps to prevent the mixture freezing too hard. If you do not use an artificial sweetener in coffee, you will not need to add any to the sorbet!

Drinks

When on a slimming diet it is particularly important to maintain a good intake of fluids and long, refreshing drinks can also help to ward off hunger pangs! A blender is invaluable in creating vitamin-packed fruit and vegetable cocktails, or whisking nutritious drinks such as Breakfast in a Glass which can equally well be drunk at other times of the day. More and more people are choosing low-alcohol or non-alcoholic drinks at parties and fruit cups and punches like Summer Cup and Tea, Rum and Orange Punch are always popular with slimmers, drivers and the health-conscious.

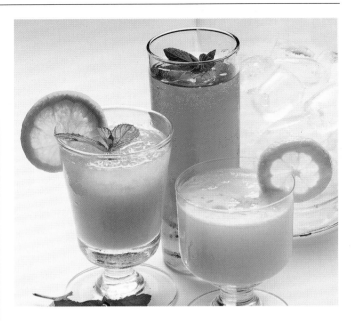

261 | Lemon and Limeade

Preparation time
10 minutes, plus chilling

Serves 4

Calories
4 per portion

You will need
juice of 3 limes
juice of 2 lemons
peeled rind of 1 lime
peeled rind of 2 lemons
1.2 litres/2 pints mineral water
1 teaspoon angostura bitters (optional)
artificial sweetener, to taste

Combine all the ingredients except the artificial sweetener and chill for 2 hours. Taste and add artificial sweetener if necessary. Serve in tall glasses.

262 | Green Summer Cooler

Preparation time
5 minutes

Serves 4

Calories
25 per portion

You will need
4 tablespoons crème de menthe
crushed ice
1.2 litres/2 pints sparkling mineral water
mint sprigs, to garnish

Put a teaspoonful of the crème de menthe in the bottom of four tall glasses. Add a little crushed ice, top up with sparkling mineral water and serve immediately garnished with mint sprigs.

Cook's Tip

Store citrus fruit in the crisper drawer of the refrigerator. Always taste any food or drink after it has been chilled as this can affect the amount of flavouring or sweetening required.

Cook's Tip

You can use a special gadget which crushes ice in a lidded container or put ice cubes in a strong polythene bag and smash them with a wooden mallet. There are also crushed ice dispensers in some large supermarkets.

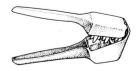

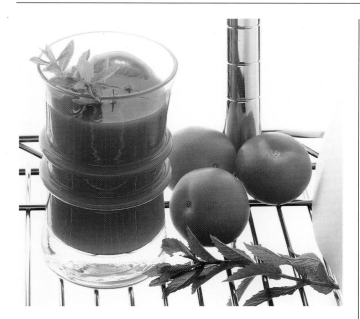

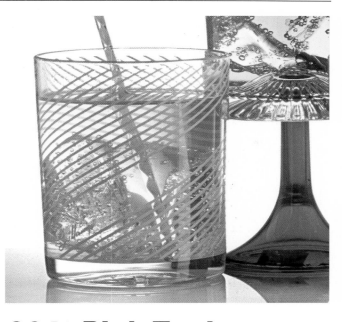

263 | Tomato Juice

Preparation time
15 minutes, plus
chilling

Serves 4

Calories
26 per portion

You will need
500 g/1¼ lb ripe tomatoes, peeled
   and roughly chopped
1 teaspoon salt
1 teaspoon lemon juice
1 teaspoon soft brown sugar
1 teaspoon Worcestershire sauce
300 ml/½ pint water
1 teaspoon tomato purée
pepper

For the garnish
4 mint sprigs
4 lemon slices

Put all the ingredients, with pepper to taste, in a blender and blend for 30 seconds. Rub through a sieve to remove the seeds, then chill for about 2 hours.

Pour the tomato juice into glasses and garnish with mint sprigs and lemon slices to serve.

264 | Pink Tonic

Preparation time
2 minutes

Serves 4

Calories
6 per portion

You will need
1 litre/1¾ pints low-calorie tonic
   water
few drops of angostura bitters
ice cubes

Divide the tonic water between four glasses and stir a few drops of angostura bitters into each glass. Add ice cubes and serve immediately.

Cook's Tip

If you have a surplus of ripe tomatoes at the peak of their growing season, turn some into tomato juice. You can vary the flavour subtly by using celery or garlic salt.

Cook's Tip

Make decorative ice cubes to float in summer drinks. Put a pink rose petal in each section of an ice tray, fill with water and freeze. If necessary, add a little more water to cover the petal and return to the freezer.

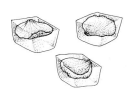

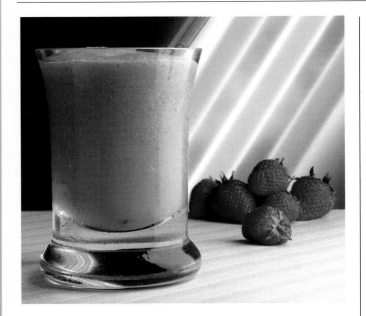

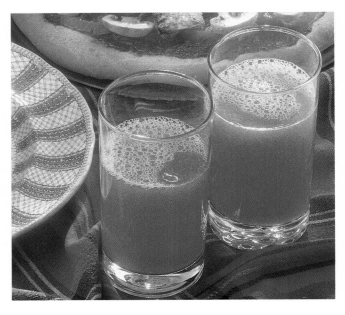

265 | *Tenderberry*

Preparation time
10 minutes

Serves 4

Calories
79 per portion

You will need
450 g/1 lb strawberries, hulled
2 tablespoons fresh orange juice
450 ml/¾ pint natural low-fat
  yogurt
crushed ice
450 ml/¾ pint low-calorie dry
  ginger ale
red food colouring
ground ginger

Reserve 4 strawberries. Put the remaining strawberries, orange juice and yogurt in a blender with some crushed ice and blend on maximum speed for 30 seconds. Divide between four tumblers. Add the dry ginger ale and a little red food colouring and stir. Sprinkle a little ginger on top and decorate each glass with one of the reserved strawberries.

266 | *Summer Cup*

Preparation time
5 minutes, plus
chilling

Cooking time
5 minutes

Serves 8

Calories
87 per portion

You will need
450 g/1 lb raspberries
1 tablespoon water
600 ml/1 pint sparkling mineral
  water
1 x 750-ml/1¼-pints bottle
  sparkling dry white wine
2 tablespoons crème de cassis

Crush the raspberries with the back of a wooden spoon and put them in a saucepan with the tablespoon of water; bring to boiling point and simmer for 3 minutes.

Cool, then combine with the other ingredients and put in an airtight container. Refrigerate overnight.

Strain the cup before serving.

Cook's Tip

Red-skinned Victoria plums can be used as an alternative to the strawberries to make an equally delicious summer drink. Try sprinkling a little cinnamon on top of each glass instead of the ground ginger.

Cook's Tip

The strained cup can be poured into a chilled vacuum flask for a picnic. As an alternative to the crème de cassis, a blackcurrant liqueur, try crème de framboise, a raspberry liqueur.

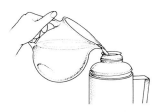

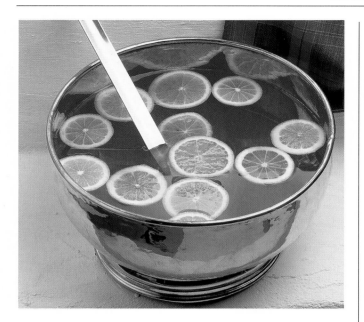

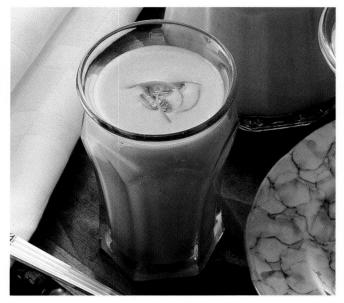

267 | Tea, Rum and Orange Punch

Preparation time
20 minutes

Serves 8

Calories
94 per portion

You will need
10 oranges
2 litres/3 ½ pints hot tea, not too
   strong
2 lemons
1 cinnamon stick
120 ml/4 fl oz dark rum
artificial sweetener, to taste

Peel a very thin layer of skin from one of the oranges and steep it in the freshly made hot tea. Squeeze the juice out of all the fruit except one half orange and one half lemon. Strain both juices and heat gently with the cinnamon stick.

Slice the half orange and half lemon as thinly as possible and soak the slices in the rum. When the orange and lemon juice reaches boiling point stir it into the tea, add the rum with the fruit slices. Taste, and stir in artificial sweetener to taste, if liked. Remove the rind and cinnamon stick before serving.

268 | Breakfast in a Glass

Preparation time
15 minutes, plus
soaking and chilling

Cooking time
10-12 minutes

Serves 4

Calories
266 per portion

You will need
75 g/3 oz porridge oats
300 ml/½ pint skimmed milk
2 large cooking apples, peeled,
   cored and chopped
grated rind of 1 orange
juice of 2 oranges
300 ml/½ pint buttermilk, chilled
2 tablespoons honey
2 eggs
2 tablespoons jumbo oats

Put the porridge oats and skimmed milk in a bowl, cover and leave to soak overnight in the refrigerator.

Put the apple, orange rind, reserving a few strands, and orange juice into a small saucepan, bring to the boil and simmer for 10 minutes, or until the apple is tender. Set aside to cool, then chill overnight.

The following morning put the porridge oats, milk, apple, buttermilk, honey and eggs in a blender and liquidize.

Divide the drink between four glasses, sprinkle the jumbo oats and reserved orange rind on top and serve immediately.

Cook's Tip

Tea may be considered the national drink of Britain but it is only rarely used as an ingredient. A flowery orange pekoe would be a particularly suitable tea to use in this punch. Alternatively, try one of the mild herbal teas.

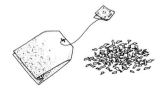

Cook's Tip

If you and your family are tempted to skip breakfast in the rush to get ready in the morning, try serving this nutritious drink. It will help to stave off those mid-morning hunger pangs.

Index